Diagno... ... ...
C ... l
... ...s

Diagnosing and Treating Computer-Related Vision Problems

James E. Sheedy, OD, PhD

Associate Professor
Ohio State University College of Optometry
Columbus, Ohio

Peter G. Shaw-McMinn, OD

Assistant Professor of Clinical Science
Southern California College of Optometry
Fullerton, California
Benedict Professor in Practice Management
University of Houston College of Optometry
Houston, Texas

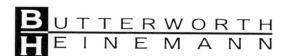

An imprint of Elsevier Science
Amsterdam   Boston   London   New York   Oxford   Paris
San Diego   San Francisco   Singapore   Sydney   Tokyo

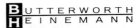

An imprint of Elsevier Science

200 Wheeler Road
Burlington, MA 01803

Notice

Optometry is an ever-changing field. Standard safety precautions must be followed, but as new research and clinical experience broaden our knowledge, changes in treatment and drug therapy may become necessary or appropriate. Readers are advised to check the most current product information provided by the manufacturer of each drug to be administered to verify the recommended dose, the method and duration of administration, and contraindications. It is the responsibility of the treating physician, relying on experience and knowledge of the patient, to determine dosages and the best treatment for each individual patient. Neither the Publisher nor the author assume any liability for any injury and/or damage to persons or property arising from this publication.

The Publisher

Library of Congress Cataloging-in-Publication Data

Sheedy, James E.
    Diagnosing and treating computer-related vision problems / James E. Sheedy, Peter G. Shaw-McMinn.
        p. cm.
    Includes bibliographical references.
    ISBN 0-7506-7404-0
    1. Vision disorders. 2. Video display terminals—Health aspects. 3. Computer users—Health and hygiene. 4. Eyestrain. I. Shaw-McMinn, Peter G. II. Title.

RE91 .S447 2003
617.7—dc21

                                                                          2002026269

Publishing Director: Linda Duncan
Managing Editor: Christie Hart

SSC/MVY
Printed in the United States of America.

Last digit is the print number: 9 8 7 6 5 4 3 2 1

Preface

We were serving on the Vision Council of America Computer Vision Task force when it became apparent that a book was necessary on the topic. Statistics were shared that demonstrated that the average patient seen in our offices was a computer user. Computer use had given rise to a host of symptoms requiring a broad approach. Many of these symptoms related to the eyes but were also contributed to by ergonomic factors.

The question to be answered was, How can eye care professionals provide comfortable vision to their computer-using patients? This led us to answer other questions such as, What office systems must be modified or added to provide proper vision care to this population? What knowledge and skills are necessary for doctors, opticians, and staff to be able to provide the necessary vision care? How can the general public be educated as to what is available to assist in concentrating for long hours on computer monitors?

This book provides all the information that any eye care professional needs to provide optimal care for computer-using patients— and to develop a specialty in this large and growing area of eye care.

An exceptional feature of this book is that it contains accurate scientific information about vision, the eye, and ergonomics; practical information about examining the eyes; and detailed information about practice management and marketing these services to your patients. We blended our respective scientific and management strengths, producing a book that is firmly based in visual science, providing the scientific underpinnings for this area of care and also giving a road map for implementing this specialty care in your practice. Almost every chapter ends with Action Items to assist you in providing vision care to the computer user.

The underlying causes of eye and vision problems can be diagnosable eye disorders or workplace ergonomic factors, or both; both are thoroughly covered in this book. This book begins with an overview of the vision and eye problems of computer users (Chapter 1) and then quickly provides a detailed discussion about how to position your practice so that patients know that you are an expert at treating their computer-related problems (Chapter 2).

Patient symptoms can be used to guide the practitioner to the most likely diagnoses, whether they are eye related or workplace related. The most common ocular conditions (refractive errors, accommodative disorders, binocular vision disorders, presbyopia, and dry eyes) are covered in Chapters 3–7. Each chapter includes a review of the pertinent literature. Research is applied to clinical evaluation, diagnosis, and management. Spectacles, contact lenses, and pharmaceutical prescribing options are covered.

Aspects of the work environment, such as lighting, display characteristics, screen reflections, and work placement (Chapters 8–11), can be significant in causing or contributing to patient symptoms. Symptom resolution can be greatly enhanced with the in-office techniques presented in these chapters. As with the vision topics, the scientific basis of these visual ergonomic topics provides background for specific clinical diagnosis and management. Chapter 12 explains how an eye care practitioner can serve as an on-site vision consultant to meet company eye care and ergonomic needs.

The last two chapters (Chapters 13 and 14) of the book include considerable information about expanding your practice with this specialty. Chapter 13 covers the unique issues of children and low vision patients at computers. Chapter 14 provides the information and tools to market your newfound specialty to your patients.

This book is the first written to prepare you and your practice for the treatment of patients with vision problems at computers. Use it to increase patient satisfaction and provide better vision care for your computer-using patients.

J.E.S.
P.G.S-M.

Acknowledgments

What a pleasure to be able to share my experiences with you through this book! Patients with problems related to computer usage are not only a large segment of those seen by most eye care practices, but also are challenging to diagnose and treat. I have spent a considerable portion of my career studying what has come to be known as *computer vision syndrome* (CVS).* These endeavors have led to professional exchanges and relationships with colleagues in a wide range of disciplines because the study of CVS necessarily leads to an interface between eye care and workplace ergonomics. I am particularly pleased that my friend and colleague, Peter Shaw-McMinn, has been able to join me in this effort. His understanding of office management and implementation of eye care has greatly enhanced the applicability of the lessons in this book.

As a beginning faculty member at Ohio State University in the late 1970s, I accepted my teaching assignments with resignation: two courses on lighting, industrial vision, public health, monocular sensory processes, and the eye as an optical instrument. My course topics did not exactly inspire interest on the part of students, but, along with my graduate studies in visual comfort, what a springboard they provided for involvement in CVS! The Ohio State University College of Optometry had a long history of expertise in workplace vision, largely through the work of Glenn A. Fry, my primary mentor and role model, and H. Richard Blackwell, a world leader in lighting, under whom I also studied.

When I moved to the University of California, Berkeley, in the early 1980s, I was immediately confronted with large numbers of computer

---

*Use of the term *computer vision syndrome* (CVS) has caused some controversy. We fully acknowledge that it is an atypical use of "syndrome" and that CVS per se is not a diagnosable condition. Instead, CVS is an umbrella that covers the numerous diagnostic conditions—eye and environment related—that are covered in this book. The value of CVS is as a communication term to the public. It is an easy moniker to communicate and refer to the various vision and eye problems experienced by computer users, which are, by the way, the most frequent health-related problems of computer users. The term CVS was originally used in the public relations campaign of a manufacturer. It has gained relatively widespread acceptance in the public domain—a fact that supports the need for the term. CVS is useful in communicating the public health issues surrounding vision at computers.

users with eye-related problems and a liberal political environment that valued answers and solutions. The idea for establishing a special treatment clinic for computer-using patients came out of a conversation with Ian Bailey, a brilliant colleague with a big heart and a taste for wine, and Sam Berman, a friend and colleague who further advanced my understanding of lighting. The VDT Eye Clinic, as it was originally known, was the first of its kind and served as a centerpiece for my work on what eventually became known as CVS. I worked hard to prepare myself while at Ohio State University but with no idea of what I was preparing for. In California, I happened to be the right person at the right time.

The multidisciplinary nature of CVS has enabled me to establish collegial and, often, deeper relationships with a wide range of individuals. Aside from those already mentioned, the following people have had the greatest impact on my thoughts: Rolland von Stroh and Bill Grenewalt from OCLI; Tom van Overbeek from Cornerstone Imaging; David Rempel and Ira Janowicz from the University of California, San Francisco; Tom Armstrong from the University of Michigan; Wanda Smith from Hewlett Packard; Cynthia Purvis from Compaq; Bengt Knave from the International Commission on Occupational Health; Bruno Piccoli from the University of Milan; Tom Albin and Sharon Middendorf from 3M; Mike White; Judy Leese and Bill Stumpf from Herman Miller; Eileen Vollowitz from Back Designs; Bill Marras from Ohio State University; Cosmo Salibello and Jon Torrey from PRIO; Laura Stock from the Labor Occupational Health Program; Todd Riley and Don Yee from Vision Service Plan; Mike Morris from SOLA; Rod Tahran from Essilor; Joe Bruneni from the Optical Laboratories Association; and Jeffrey Anshel and Steve Glasser, a couple of colleagues with whom I have worked closely for many years.

I would be completely remiss if I did not also acknowledge a couple of wonderful women in my personal life without whom the circumstances that led to writing this book would not have occurred. Patty was a wonderful support during my academic development at Ohio State University and caused me to move to California. Debora gave me the ability to develop and appreciate fullness in life, both professionally and personally. I thank them both.

J.E.S.

Jim has acknowledged many of the individuals who have provided expertise, allowing us to write this book. In addition, I would like to thank Gary Moss, who has been a friend and colleague sharing his marketing theory with me through the years. Gary, I have always found your high energy motivating. Thanks. Most of all, I've got to thank Jim Sheedy for giving me the opportunity to contribute to the book. Jim is a pleasure to work with. He thinks rationally and is creative, both at work and play. I'll never forget the weekend we locked ourselves in the hotel room and hammered out the final manuscript! It was one of the most enjoyable experiences of my life. You are the greatest, Jim!

I must also acknowledge the individual who probably has taught me the most about computer use. Everyone should have a resource to lean on when using computer hardware and software to the fullest. My resource has set up wireless networks in my office and at home. He maintains our Web sites and assists in any computer-related endeavors. He was only 10 years old when he began educating his dear ol' dad. At the time of this printing, he has become my 15-year-old Informational Technology expert. Thanks Lysle for your technical and intellectual assistance in writing this book. Thanks for being patient with an old guy! And thanks to the rest of my family for putting up with all the time spent e-mailing back and forth to Jim and our wonderful editors, Christie Hart and Brooke Begin.

P.G.S-M.

Contents

1
Computer Vision Syndrome

Computers are used by 100 million people in the United States at their jobs every day (U.S. Bureau of Labor Statistics). Since 1999, according to the National Center for Education Statistics, 95% of schools and 63% of all classrooms have had Internet access. On a typical day, even children 2–5 years of age spend an average of 27 minutes on a computer (Lucile Packard Foundation, 2001). Computers have become the primary medium through which we receive information—and we receive it through our eyes and visual system.

Vision- and eye-related problems at computer displays* are very common and have collectively been named *computer vision syndrome* (CVS) by the American Optometric Association. The prevalence of eye symptoms among computer users ranges from 25% to 93%, as reported by various investigators (Thompson, 1998). Clearly, a large percentage of computer workers experience eye symptoms. This results in a large number of computer users seeking eye care.

Surveys of optometrists (Sheedy, 1992; Nilsen and Salibello, 1997) show that approximately one out of six primary-care eye examinations is given in the United States primarily because of vision and eye-related problems at computers. The cost of these eye examinations and special computer glasses is nearly $2 billion—this is a significant health care issue and a significant part of most eye care practices.

In addition to having numerous patients with symptoms of CVS, the treatment of patients can be quite challenging to the eye care practitioner. There are many sources of CVS symptoms and corresponding treatment choices. Each patient has a different set of eyes and

---

*Computer displays have commonly been referred to as video display terminals, but this term refers to older displays that are no longer used. Hence, the term is not emphasized in this book.

different workstation circumstances. The challenge of the examining doctor is to identify the possible causes of symptoms and design an appropriate treatment plan. Providing excellent computer vision care improves patient quality of life; it can also help a practice to grow.

The purposes of this book are as follows:

- Provide the eye care practitioner with the necessary information to understand the visual and work environment causes of CVS
- Identify the methods of optimally treating the eyes and modifying the work environment
- Provide methods by which this can be integrated into an eye care practice
- Provide the information to become expert in CVS and to build a practice with this knowledge

Computer Vision Syndrome Background

Vision problems at computers result in visual inefficiencies and cause eye-related symptoms among computer workers. The primary symptoms of CVS are listed in Box 1-1 (Sheedy, 1992). All of the symptoms listed in Box 1-1 have long been recognized and documented as being associated with demanding visual work—especially demanding near visual work. Secretaries, accountants, bookkeepers, draftsmen, and others with demanding near visual jobs have commonly experienced many of these symptoms. However, there are many aspects of computer work that make it considerably more visually demanding than other near tasks.

The causes of CVS are a combination of individual visual problems and poor visual ergonomics. The symptoms occur whenever the visual demands of the task exceed the visual abilities of the individual. For example, many individuals have marginal vision disorders such as uncorrected refractive errors, accommodative disorders, or binocular vision disorders that do not cause symptoms when performing less demanding visual tasks. Likewise, there are numerous aspects of the computer display and its work environment, such as lighting, reflections, poor display quality, flicker, and workstation arrangement, that can make computer

> **Box 1-1**
>
> The primary vision- and eye-related complaints among computer users are as follows:
>
> - Eyestrain (sore eyes or eye fatigue)
> - Headache
> - Near blurred vision
> - Slowness in changing the focus of the eyes
> - Blur in the distance after near work
> - Glare (light) sensitivity
> - Eye irritation (burning, dryness, redness)
> - Contact lens discomfort
> - Neck and shoulder pain
> - Back pain

work a more demanding visual task than others; therefore, more individuals are put beyond their threshold for experiencing symptoms.

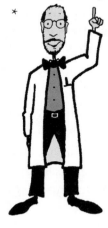

The computer task is particularly visually demanding and, therefore, causes symptoms in patients who would not have any difficulties with less demanding vision tasks. This makes diagnosing and treating CVS particularly difficult for the eye care practitioner. Two surveys of optometrists showed they were significantly less able to arrive confidently at a diagnosis and treatment for patients with computer-related problems compared to other patients (Sheedy, 1992; Nilsen and Salibello, 1997). There are two likely reasons for this greater diagnostic uncertainty for computer-using patients: (1) The vision disorders require more testing and more aggressive diagnosis

---

*Doctor Ergo is a registered trademark owned by Dr. James E. Sheedy. Images of Doctor Ergo appear throughout this book. Dr. Sheedy retains all rights in the name and the images of Doctor Ergo.

for computer-using patients because of the greater visual demands of the task, and (2) many of the problems are caused or contributed to by workplace ergonomic conditions. The visual problems of computer-using patients are more difficult to resolve than those of other patients.

The vision problems of computer users are very real and very prevalent, and most of the causative factors are known. The visual symptoms can largely be resolved with proper management of the environment and by providing proper visual care (Aaras et al., 1998). A high degree of success (Sheedy and Parsons, 1990) has been attained at resolving patient symptoms in a clinical setting by applying the following two-pronged approach:

1. Careful diagnosis and treatment of visual conditions that cause CVS symptoms
2. In-office diagnosis and management of workstation ergonomic deficiencies

For some patients, it is clearly a specific visual disorder that is responsible for the symptoms; for other patients, it is more clearly a particular environmental condition that is causing the symptoms. In many other patients it is less clear. Sometimes, a particular patient has two or more very marginal visual disorders and also has two or three problems in the workstation environment. In such situations, it is best to resolve all of the causative conditions and factors.

About This Book

This book addresses the eye-related and environmental factors that cause visual problems and other symptoms for computer users and suggests methods for implementing diagnosis and management of both into an eye care practice.

Chapter 2 focuses on making your practice patient friendly to computer users. Positioning your practice properly through office design and office policies will allow effective communication with the computer-using patient. Immediately upon entering the practice, patients should recognize that the office is geared to serve their needs.

By the time the patients have gone through the segments of a typical patient visit, they will be enthusiastic supporters of the practice.

Chapter 3 focuses on the presenting symptoms of CVS and how they can efficiently lead to the diagnosis. History forms and questionnaires are provided to aid the assistant or technician in responding properly to the patient's concerns. Chapters 4–7 discuss the primary vision and eye conditions that cause symptoms and how they can be most effectively diagnosed and treated. These include refractive errors, accommodative disorders, binocular vision problems, presbyopia, and dry eye.

Chapters 8–11 discuss the key workplace factors that cause CVS. These include lighting, reflections, computer display, and workstation arrangement. In-office methods of evaluating and treating each of these workplace factors are outlined. Chapter 12 provides the information needed to perform workplace evaluations as an eye care consultant. Chapter 13 discusses special issues about children working at computers, as well as low vision patients at computers.

The final chapter explains how to develop a marketing plan for an eye care practice in the area of CVS.

References

Aaras A, Horgen G, Bjorset H, et al. Musculoskeletal, visual and psychosocial stress in VDU operators before and after multidisciplinary ergonomic interventions. Appl Ergon 1998;29(5):335–354.

Nilsen E, Salibello C. Survey of U.S. optometrists regarding prevalence and treatment of visual stress symptoms. HCI International '97. Proceedings of the 7th International Conference on Human-Computer Interaction 1997, San Francisco, California. Boston: Elsevier Science, 1997;24–30.

Lucile Packard Foundation. Children and computer technology: issues and ideas or the edition entitled Children and Computer Technology, 2001. Children and Computer Technology: Issues and Ideas. Available at: http://www.futureofchildren.org. Accessed May 2, 2002.

Sheedy JE. Vision problems at video display terminals: a survey of optometrists. J Am Optom Assoc 1992;63:687–692.

Sheedy JE, Parsons SP. The video display terminal eye clinic: clinical report. Optom Vis Sci 1990;67(8):622–626.

Thompson WD. Eye problems and visual display terminals—the facts and fallacies. Ophthalmic Physiol Opt 1998;18(2):111–119.

2
Positioning Your Practice to Care for Computer-User Patients

Sometimes eye care professionals forget what it is like to think as a patient. Research on how patients evaluate services demonstrates that they make their decisions based on many "little things," as opposed to one or two large factors. The following five main characteristics of service delivery that contribute to patients' overall perceptions about quality are referred to as *RATER* (Zeithami et al., 1990):

1. *Reliability*—the ability to perform the promised service dependably and accurately
2. *Assurance*—the staff's knowledge, courtesy, and ability to convey credibility, trustworthiness, and competence
3. *Tangibles*—the physical appearance of the facility, equipment, staff, and communication materials
4. *Empathy*—caring, individualized attention; understanding the patient's concerns and situation; and effective communication with the patient
5. *Responsiveness*—willingness to assist patients and provide prompt service without patients experiencing obstacles or an inability to gain access to your services

Of the five stated components of service quality, reliability is an outcome, whereas the other four are part of the service delivery process. The last three (tangibles, empathy, responsiveness) are often the direct results of employee performance (Parasuraman et al., 1991).

This chapter focuses on making your practice computer-user patient friendly by attending to these desirable service qualities.

Computer-User Patient-Friendly Office

Positioning your practice properly through office design and office policies allows you to communicate effectively with the computer-user patient. Immediately on entering the practice, the patient recognizes that the office is geared to serve his or her needs. By the time the patient has gone through the segments of a typical patient visit, he or she is an enthusiastic supporter of the practice. You benefit from the enthusiastic computer-user patient recommending you to coworkers and friends.

Positioning the Practice before Patients Come for Appointments

A computer-using patient will draw certain conclusions about how he or she is treated in the practice. These "moments of truth" (Moss and Shaw-McMinn, 2001; Shaw-McMinn, 2001) begin with the telephone call to make an appointment. An on-hold message can begin the process of educating the patient by saying,

---

"Dr. Gates and his staff use the latest technology to improve your vision and lifestyle. Many of our patients are now using computers at work and play. Dr. Gates has the latest equipment for examining the visual system to ensure that computer use does not result in symptoms and poor performance. He may prescribe eye exercises or lens products that are designed specifically for computer users. . . ."

Because a large percentage of patients calling for an examination are computer users, it makes sense for your receptionist to make a statement regarding computer usage when scheduling the first appointment:

"Mrs. Smith, how many hours a day do you use a computer? Six? Dr. Gates and his staff will design an examination specifically for taking care of your needs, including advising you on using the computer. There are many new services and products that relieve much of the eyestrain caused by computer use."

The patient now has the idea that the office he or she has chosen knows how to care for his or her computer-using needs. Some offices reinforce this notion by mailing a history form to the patient before the visit. The mailing of information before the scheduled appointment often generates enthusiasm. The patient looks forward to experiencing the examination and learning what can be done to improve his or her vision and comfort. An example of a mailing before the examination can include a cover letter indicating purpose, description of office and staff, services and products provided, brochures, and the history form with a self-addressed stamped envelope.

Showing patients that you use computer technology yourself indicates to them that you are computer savvy and may understand the problems they experience. At the very least, it shows you are high tech. An example of this would be to have your own Web site with the capability to schedule appointments over the Internet. Because the patient is computer literate, browsing the Web site should be easy for him or her and more convenient than calling an office. On your Web site, you can emphasize computer vision care and provide information on tests specifically for computer users or products that are available for computer users (Figure 2-1).

A previsit history form can easily be downloaded from the Web site and information entered before the appointment. Questions concerning matters such as distance of the computer screen from their eyes indicate a concern on the part of the doctor. Patients will get a good "feeling" about the office before they have even entered it.

Any external marketing you do should include the mention of your ability to treat computer vision syndrome (CVS). Information from

Welcome To
Woodcrest Vision Center
"High tech vision for high tech computer-users"

The professionals in our office provide the latest in high tech instrumentation, services and products to enable the computer-user to work long hours comfortably. Our mission is to protect your future vision and improve your life.

Virginia Martinez   Jessica Seymour
Mary Shaw-McMinn   Tammy Beishline
Michael Kobayashi, OD Peter Shaw-McMinn, OD

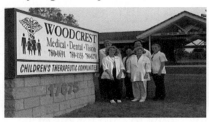

Links

W elcome
C omputer-user Vision Exam
C omputer-user History Form
S chedule An Appointment
P roducts
S ervices
L ibary

Office Hours:

mon	9:00AM-7:00PM
tues	9:00AM-8:00PM
wed	9:00AM-5:00PM
thu	9:00AM-5:00PM
fri	9:00AM-3:00PM
sat	Closed
sun	Closed

FIGURE 2-1. Web site.

outside the practice also serves to set the proper image in the minds of your patients before they have even entered the practice!

Positioning the Practice through Computers in the Reception Area

When the patient enters the office, you have another opportunity to demonstrate that it is prepared to care for computer users. A practice that is computer literate has computers distributed throughout the office for use by staff. I've heard patients comment about their doctors' offices by saying, "His office didn't even use computers! I wonder how far behind they are in their doctor stuff?" (This was a 70-year-old lady saying this!) Computer-using patients expect to see computers in a practice; place them so they are visible to the patient.

You can surpass patients' expectations by having computer workstations available for them to use in the reception room (Figure 2-2).

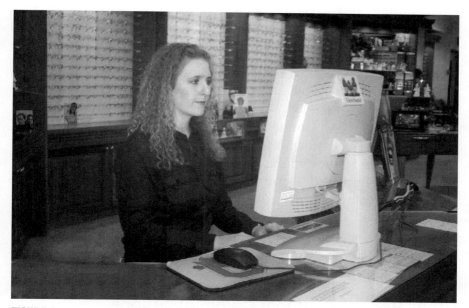

FIGURE 2-2. Photo of workstation for patients in reception room.

This demonstrates a patient-friendly attitude and also doubles as an examination procedure by allowing you to observe them at work on the computer. Computer workstations hooked to a digital subscriber line (DSL) connection networked to several computers indicates to the patient that this office is indeed computer-user friendly. While waiting for the doctor, patients have the option of getting on the Internet and checking e-mail, sending messages, surfing the Web for information, or completing their work for the day.

The patient workstations also give the office an idea of how the patient may be operating at his or her own workstation. Does the patient blink frequently? Is the patient's posture unusual? What is the patient's working distance? Prescribed treatments such as screen filters or adjustments in working distance and visual axis angle can be demonstrated at the workstation after the examination. Providing computers for use by patients definitely sets you apart as a computer-user friendly office. Patients surfing the Internet while waiting for family members to complete their examinations will be heard to exclaim, "You're done already?" "Already" may be 45–60 minutes. Computer-using patients do not mind waiting if they are able to use the computer in the reception room to complete tasks they are interested in.

You can network a series of computers to your office DSL by using a Linksys router. You can attach three computers via a wireless as well as a serial port hardwired computer. Connect your DSL modem or cable to Linksys EtherFast Wireless AP + Cable/DSL Router (model number BEFW11S4). Connect a Linksys Instant Wireless USB (universal serial bus) Network Adapter (model number WUSB11) to the USB serial port in the computers you wish to network with the computer that is connected to your modem and router. (You need a USB port in your computer; if you do not have one, you can add it for as little as $10.00). Configure the system and you have a wireless network so your patients can surf the Internet while waiting. For more information, see http://www.linksys.com.

Other Reception Room Communications

In addition to the computers in the office reception area, other marketing techniques may be useful for educating the patient. Take-one boxes may be strategically placed with brochures on lenses designed for presbyopic computer users, such as the Interview lens by Essilor or the Access lens by SOLA. Counter cards are often available from labs that hold brochures on possible treatments the doctor may prescribe. For example, 3M provides a counter-card display with a computer monitor and take-one brochures that say, "Do you experience eyestrain, eye fatigue, or glare-related headaches due to computer monitor use?" A picture of a monitor with an eye on the screen with glare is beneath the statement, followed by, "If you answered yes, read on for ways to improve your viewing comfort." The brochure goes on to give tips for reducing eyestrain, the first tip being "Get an eye examination." The brochure is for a computer filter that reduces glare (3M Optical Systems).

Your business card should include the office Web site address and e-mail address. Some business cards act as a mini-brochure by including a logo, theme, and services provided, such as computer vision examinations. Some offices include computerized patient history software such as Status View. It is a 5-minute touch-screen patient self-interviewing system that asks patients lifestyle questions and questions you would expect to be asked in a history. Computer users feel particularly comfortable on the system. It gives a "high-tech" appearance to the office. For more information, see http://www.statusview.com.

A computer-user–friendly program that recently came on the market for use with your patients is EyeMaginations. EyeMaginations is a computer program multimedia suite of three-dimensional animations that educate patients in all eye care areas (i.e., anatomy, dispensing, pathology, clinical procedures, and refractive errors). Without a doctor or staff saying a word, patients have explained conditions, options, or what to look out for in their eye health. This high-tech tool is a valuable time saver that "raises the bar" on the way we, eye care professionals, educate our patients. It includes an excellent presentation on CVS. For more information, see http://www.eyemaginations.com.

A reception area with magazines about computers also shows that you are interested in computers. Magazines such as *PC Magazine, PC World, Byte Magazine, Computer World,* and *Computer Edge* keep the patient interested while waiting for an examination room to clear. You can receive the last two magazines at no charge. For more information, you can access their Web sites.

Pictures on the wall showing computer-using patients or testimonials from satisfied patients can go a long way in developing the image of an office that knows how to care for computer users and their problems. Testimonials can be powerful marketing tools. The hallways leading to the executive offices of the meeting department at Disneyland reveal one testimonial after another. When patients have nice things to say, ask them if you can have it typed up on their stationery and framed on the wall—most patients feel honored.

A glassed-in reception area with the latest in computerized video-game machines such as Playstation and Nintendo will keep children happy as they wait for the doctor. The glassed-in area muffles the noise from the sound effects of the games. You will find that children are anxious to come to the office and actually look forward to playing computer games in the reception area (Figure 2-3).

Having the latest palm pilot or minicomputer may impress the computer user that you are up on the latest computer technology.

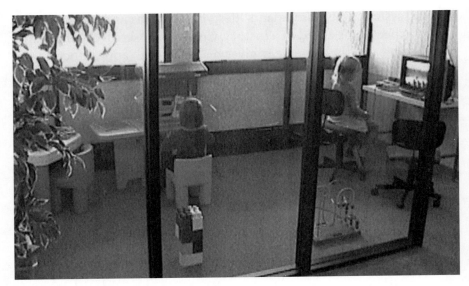

FIGURE 2-3. Photo of children's reception area.

They will naturally deduce that if you are up on the latest computer technology, you will probably be up on the latest eye care technology. The new flat LCD (liquid crystal display) monitors also make the high-tech statement. Patients will see the monitors and wish they had them. All these small things add together to position the office as the best place for a computer user to obtain eye care! They contribute to the RATER perceptions our patients value.

Office Forms

Your "welcome to the office" materials, patient history form, examination form, and receipts can all be changed to reflect your interest in computer-user patients.

History Form

Some doctors use a history form specific to CVS, whereas others simply add a few questions to their present form. An example of questions to add follows:

Do you wish to receive electronic updates on the latest developments
   in vision and ocular health-related issues? _____
E-mail address _____
How many hours a day do you use a computer? _____
How long before your eyes grow tired or get irritated? _____

These questions show patients you are up on the latest technology
(e-mail and perhaps a Web site) and encourage them to think
about whether eye discomfort can be related to computer use.
Many patients still do not make the connection, or they assume it
is normal to have symptoms after 1 or 2 hours on the computer
(Shaw-McMinn, 2001). An example of a history form specific to
computer users developed by a CVS doctor is illustrated in Figure
2-4.

Examination Form

A typical examination for a computer user may include testing for
all visual skills and eye conditions. Because patients of all ages are
using computers today, any possible procedure can be important
for your patient. As our older patients begin to use computers
more frequently, many pathologic conditions must be addressed in
playing a role in computer-use comfort. Figure 2-5 shows an
examination form that may be used for computer users. Note the
label "Computer-User Examination Form" at the top. Patients will
notice the label and discern that you administer an examination
tailored for their particular concerns. Providing an examination
specific to computer users sets you apart from other eye care
practitioners.

Treatment Routing Slip

Many doctors use a slip to indicate the treatment by checking off
options and handing it to the optician with the words, "Please demonstrate the following to Ms. Rom. Ms. Rom, Jennifer will show you
the prescribed treatment I explained to you and set up a follow-up
appointment." Figure 2-6 is a sample routing slip.

CVS Doctors History Form

Name_____   Date_____

Symptom Assessment

Please circle whether or not (**Y** or **N**) you experience each of the following symptoms. For each **Y** answer, circle the appropriate number to identify the severity of the symptom.

Y N	**Eyestrain**												
			Mild				Moderate						Severe
	If YES, rate:	Severity	0	1	2	3	4	5	6	7	8	9	10

Comments:

Y N	**Tired eyes**												
			Mild				Moderate						Severe
	If YES, rate:	Severity	0	1	2	3	4	5	6	7	8	9	10

Comments:

Y N	**Headache**												
			Mild				Moderate						Severe
	If YES, rate:	Severity	0	1	2	3	4	5	6	7	8	9	10

Comments:

Y N	**Irritated or sore eyes**												
			Mild				Moderate						Severe
	If YES, rate:	Severity	0	1	2	3	4	5	6	7	8	9	10

Comments:

Y N	**Dry eyes**												
			Mild				Moderate						Severe
	If YES, rate:	Severity	0	1	2	3	4	5	6	7	8	9	10

Comments:

Y N	**Lighting or glare discomfort**												
			Mild				Moderate						Severe
	If YES, rate:	Severity	0	1	2	3	4	5	6	7	8	9	10

Comments:

Y N	**Blurred vision**												
			Mild				Moderate						Severe
	If YES, rate:	Severity	0	1	2	3	4	5	6	7	8	9	10

Comments:

Y N	**Neck or shoulder ache**												
			Mild				Moderate						Severe
	If YES, rate:	Severity	0	1	2	3	4	5	6	7	8	9	10

Comments:

Y N	**Back ache**												
			Mild				Moderate						Severe
	If YES, rate:	Severity	0	1	2	3	4	5	6	7	8	9	10

Comments:

Y N	**Hand or wrist ache**												
			Mild				Moderate						Severe
	If YES, rate:	Severity	0	1	2	3	4	5	6	7	8	9	10

Comments:

FIGURE 2-4. Computer vision syndrome (CVS) doctor patient history form.

COMPUTER-USER EXAMINATION FORM

Name _____ Address _____ Phone _____

Review of computer-related signs and symptoms

Rx _____ Computer distance _____

Date	far va s Rx	c Rx	near va s Rx	c Rx

Ks _____

Ret. _____ Near Ret. _____

Subj. _____ va _____ Near Subj. _____

PR phoria	BI/BO	Stereo	Supp	Fix disparity
near add	va	PP phoria	BI	BO
NRA	PRA	AA	x-cyl	+/– 2.00

	Biomicroscopy	
PERRLA/no APD	Lashes/lids	TBUT
	Cornea	Blink rate
EOM	Conj.	Schirmer's test
CT	A.C./iris	
	Lens	Dry eye test
NPC Color vision		

T$_A$ R   L   @   VF conf R   L   VF auto   R   L   BP   /

Direct/BIO/90 D

1% tropicamide/2.5% Neo-Synephrine

Media
C/D
E
Depth
Shape
Macula/FR
A/V

Dx/Imp/Rec/RTC

FIGURE 2-5. Computer-user examination form. (AA = amplitude of accommodation; A.C. = anterior chamber; APD = afferent pupillary defect; A/V = artery/vein diameter ratio; BI/BO = base in–base out; BIO = binocular indirect ophthalmoscopy; C/D = cup-to-disk ratio; CT = cover test; Dx = diagnosis; E = esophoria; FR = foveal reflex; EOM = extraocular movements; Imp = impression; Ks = corneal curvature; NPC = near point of convergence; NRA = negative relative accommodation; PERRLA = pupils equal, round, reactive to light and accommodation; PP = punctum proximum; PR = punctum remotum; PRA = positive relative accommodation; Rec = recommendations; Ret. = retinoscopy; RTC = return call; Subj. = subjective; Supp = suppression; TBUT = tear breakup time; va = visual acuity; VF = visual field.)

Name _____ Date_____

COMPUTER SYNDROME TREATMENT PLAN		
❏ Vision therapy	❏ Ointments	❏ Lid scrubs
❏ Prism	❏ Punctal plugs	❏ Antibiotic drops
❏ Rest breaks	❏ Drink water	❏ Antiglare screen
❏ Blink training	❏ Increase humidity	❏ Consult M.D.
❏ Lubricating drops	❏ Contact lenses	re: meds
❏ Place document holder at	❏ Change monitor	❏ Avoid certain meds
same distance as monitor	distance	❏ Consult ergonomics
	❏ Allergy meds	of workstation
	❏ Medicated drops	❏ Self-evaluation of
		workstation

COMPUTER RX		
❏ Occupational progressive	❏ Non-glare coat	❏ Polycarbonate
❏ Variable focus	❏ Scratch resistant	❏ Hi-index
❏ CRT Trifocal	❏ Tint _____	❏ CR-39
❏ Executive bifocal	❏ UV 400	❏ Glass
❏ ST 35 or 45		❏ Aspheric
❏ Single vision		

Follow-up visit on _____

FIGURE 2-6. Treatment routing slip. (CRT = cathode ray tube; Rx = prescription; UV = ultraviolet.)

Examination Summary Form

Other doctors use an examination summary designed just for computer users. The use of the summary impresses many patients. It is something other doctors have not done in the past and sets you apart as a special eye care professional. Patients sometimes return with past examination summaries in hand, complete with coffee stains. They often show them to coworkers, friends, and family. A sample computer vision examination summary is illustrated in Figure 2-7.

Computer Evaluation Explanation

For those doctors who wish to receive an additional fee for a separate computer-user evaluation, an explanation of why a separate fee is nec-

COMPUTER VISION EXAM SUMMARY

Listed below is a summary of the optometric computer examination performed on the above date. Only "checked" items apply to the patient named above.

A. EYE HEALTH

❏ No disorders noted in internal or external eye structures at time of examination.

❏ Other: _____

B. VISUAL FIELD

❏ No restrictions or anomalies of the visual field were identified

❏ Other: _____

C. INTRAOCULAR PRESSURE

❏ Within normal limits at the time of the examination

❏ Other: _____

D. VISUAL ACUITY With [ ] present or [ ] no correction:

Distance: Right Eye _____ Left Eye _____ Both Eyes _____

Near: Right Eye _____ Left Eye _____ Both Eyes _____

E. REFRACTIVE STATUS

❏ Negligible refractive error

❏ Myopia (nearsightedness) of a low/moderate/high degree

❏ Hyperopia (farsightedness) of a low/moderate/high degree

❏ Astigmatism of a low/moderate/high degree

❏ Anisometropia (unequal eyes) of a moderate/high degree

❏ Other comments: _____

F. BINOCULARITY OR EYE TEAMING ABILITY

❏ Binocular skills are adequate.

❏ Binocular skills are mildly deficient.

❏ Binocular skills are markedly deficient.

❏ Strabismus (eye turn) is present.

   ❏ Esotropia (inward)

   ❏ Exotropia (outward)

   ❏ Hypertropia (upward)

❏ Other: _____

G. OCULAR MOTILITIES OR EYE TRACKING SKILLS

❏ Eye movement skills are smooth and accurate.

❏ Eye movement skills are mildly deficient.

❏ Eye movement skills are markedly deficient.

❏ Other: _____

H. ACCOMMODATION OR FOCUSING ABILITY

❏ Accommodative amplitude and facility are at expected levels.

❏ Accommodative skills are deficient.

❏ Other: _____

I. COLOR VISION

❏ Color discrimination ability is normal.

❏ Other: _____

FIGURE 2-7. Examination summary form. (O.D. = right eye; O.S. = left eye; Rx = prescription.)

J. DISPOSITION AND RECOMMENDATIONS

❑ No prescription lenses were considered necessary.

❑ No prescription change was considered necessary.

❑ Lenses have been prescribed for the following:

    ❑ Constant use

    ❑ All near work (within 24 inches)

    ❑ Computer use

    ❑ Distance viewing only

    ❑ Use at patient's discretion

    ❑ Other: _____

Visual acuity with the prescribed correction:

Distance: Right Eye _____ Left Eye _____ Both Eyes _____

Near: Right Eye _____ Left Eye _____ Both Eyes _____

❑ Vision therapy

❑ Blink training

❑ Lubricating drops/ointment _____

❑ Medication

❑ Rest breaks

❑ Adjust monitor/document distance

❑ The patient was referred for further testing:

    ❑ Computer vision evaluation

    ❑ Workstation evaluation

    ❑ Punctal plugs

    ❑ Vision training

    ❑ Contact lens

    ❑ Low vision

    ❑ Ocular pathology

    ❑ Medical consult

    ❑ Other: _____

K. CONTINUING CARE It is recommended that this patient return for his/her vision evaluation in _____ weeks _____ months _____ years

L. ADDITIONAL COMMENTS

_____
_____
_____
_____

Rx	Sphere	Cylinder	Axis	Prism	Base	Add
O.D.						
O.S.						

Type Lens	Tint/Coatings

Expiration Date _____ License No. _____

FIGURE 2-7. (*Continued*)

essary helps the patient to understand the value of your specialized service. Figure 2-8 is an example of an explanation handed to patients.

Office forms should be customized for computer users. Include computer-related vision services and products on all your office communications. Mention of computer-related offerings in your practice positions you as the eye care professional a computer user needs to see.

Positioning Your Practice in the Pretesting Room

You can communicate your expertise in computer vision by designing the proper pretesting room appearance, training the assistant on how to recognize CVS patients and to say appropriate statements to the patient, explaining the value of pretesting to computer users by use of scripts for the assistant.

Pretest Room Appearance

The room can be decorated similarly to the reception area to provide educational opportunities for the patient to learn more about services and products for computer users. Counter cards, brochures, testimonials, and certification of eye care professionals should be available to the patient to review when waiting for the assistant or technician.

Assistant Review of History and Pretesting

The assistant has an opportunity to further educate the patient during the review of the history and pretesting. An alert technician can recognize when certain treatments may be recommended by you and prepare the patient to avoid a surprise.

"Ms. Apple, I see from your history form that you use computers. Did you know that more than 100 million Americans use computers at work every day? And more than 70% of them have problems with their vision or their eyes! Dr. Gates will complete an examination customized to your needs and may prescribe eye exercises, lenses, or other treatments to make things easier on your eyes

---

THE COMPUTER VISION EVALUATION

*Understandably, many of our patients wonder what services are provided during a computer vision evaluation in addition to those provided in a general vision examination. Below is a list of **additional** services we may include during our computer vision examination. The actual procedures vary depending on the type of the computer demands, complexity of problem solving required, and individual patient characteristics. We want to do all we can to be the best provider of vision care for you. Do not hesitate to ask us any questions regarding the following:*

1. Review of computer vision history
2. Review current vision, comfort, visual demands, and patient concerns
3. Acuity at the computer screen distance
4. Retinoscopy at the working distance with PRIO computer simulator instrument
5. Subjective refraction with PRIO computer simulator instrument
6. Visual acuity with the retinoscopy finding
7. Visual acuity with the subjective finding
8. Biomicroscopy evaluation of the tear film
9. Lid evaluation with lid eversion
10. Evaluation of tear breakup time
11. Schirmer's test for tearing
12. Dry eye test
13. Blink rate measurement
14. Corneal topography
15. Color vision testing
16. Assessment of the workstation
17. Present recommendations and treatment options
18. Review patient concerns
19. Complete the computer lens prescription
20. Demonstrate the prescribed computer lenses
21. Order the computer glasses
22. Review proper use of and handling of computer glasses
23. Provide educational materials on computer vision
24. Verify proper computer glasses order delivery

As you can see, there is much that goes on during the computer vision evaluation that you may not be aware of. You can be sure that if any new technology appears that can improve our care for your eyes, we will add it to our procedures. We are dedicated to the goal for you to have "Good Vision for the Rest of Your Life!"

Ann S. Kame, O.D.	Tammy Beishline, Optician
John Hersh, O.D	Marta Frase, Optician
Clinton Wong, O.D.	Jessica Seymour, Orthoptist
Peter G. Shaw-McMinn, O.D.	Heidi Johnson, Receptionist
Shelly Burkhart, Optician	Mary Shaw-McMinn, Optician

FIGURE 2-8. Computer evaluation explanation.

when using a computer. Ms. Apple, how often do you have problems focusing? (At this point the assistant may continue investigating the frequency, duration, intensity, and related factors of the patient's signs and symptoms.)

Because you use computers, I'm going to give you a few preliminary tests to give the doctor an idea of how he can best assist you.

Stereoacuity test: "This test will give us an indication of how well you are using your eyes together at near distances, like that of a computer screen. Many people ignore one eye or strain to keep the eyes turned in for long periods of time, causing discomfort or irritation.

Visual fields: "This computerized instrument lets us know how well you see objects in your peripheral vision, like when scanning across a computer screen at work."

Lensometry: "I see from your prescription that you are using general-use lenses at your computer. There are many lenses designed specifically for use at the computer—lenses that focus at the proper computer distance with no glare and designs that allow a patient to have his or her head in a comfortable position when viewing the screen. Here is a brochure about one such possible lens that Dr. Gates may prescribe."

Assistant Script for Introducing the Doctor

After the pretesting, the assistant typically seats the patient in the examination room and may say,

---

"You'll like Dr. MacIntosh. He explains everything thoroughly, has 25 years' experience here in Woodcrest, and specializes in treating computer-user patients. Ask him about the computer lenses we discussed."

A well-trained assistant can prepare the patient for future treatment recommendations and position the practice and the doctor properly so that the computer-user patient recognizes value in the services and products he or she receives.

Positioning the Practice during the Examination

Most of positioning a computer-user practice does not directly involve the doctor. The examination is one place where the doctor can influence the perception of the computer-user patient. The doctor's appearance, demeanor, and explanations do much to convince the computer-user patient that the prescribed treatment is in his or her best interest. The examination room appearance, development of carefully worded scripts for the doctor to use, availability of visual aids for explanations, and patient education materials enable the doctor to properly position the practice.

Examination Room Appearance

In addition to being clean and well organized, the examination room can be decorated to promote computer vision, similar to the reception area or pretesting room. Certification as a doctor versed in treating CVS should be framed on the wall, as well as any awards or other recognition. You can obtain certification through http://www.CVSDoctors. com. Photographs of conditions related to CVS, such as dry eye or binocular vision problems, should be posted. Article reprints on CVS diagnosis and treatment should be kept close at hand to give the patient. Explanations of symptoms, diagnosis and treatment of binocular dysfunction, accommodative dysfunction, and convergence insufficiency can be obtained from the College of Vision Development and should be handed to the patient when appropriate. Pamphlets from the American Optometric Association, Optometric Extension Program, and the American Foundation for Vision Awareness should be available to give to the patient to reinforce the prescribed treatments. A handout to include in the examination room could be "Improving the Ergonomics of Your Computer Workstation" (see Appendix 11-1, page 202).

Explanation of Examination Procedure Scripts

Many successful doctors explain the benefits of the procedure during the examination and relate them to computer use. For example, during the pursuits and cover-test you may say,

---

"We have six muscles going to each eye. By moving them in these directions, I can isolate the muscles and see if they are working well together. Your eyes naturally assume an outward position when looking at close targets. This can cause your eyes to tire when doing near work, such as working on a computer."

Case Presentation Scripts

Often you will discover many possible causes of the CVS signs and symptoms. As with any other case, educate the patient and develop a treatment plan that covers the possible causes. Develop scripts and visual aids to assist you in conveying the need for treatment. If you've been discussing the findings with the patient all along the course of the examination, it will be no surprise for him or her to learn he or she needs assistance. Here is a sample presentation to a patient, Ms. Apple:

"Ms. Apple, I will present my examination findings to you now. Here is a picture of an eye. We have a lens on the front of the eye called the **cornea** that gives us two-thirds of our focusing power. Then we have a lens inside the eye that is connected to strings called **zonules**, which connect to muscles. This is the lens we use to change focus. Perfect vision means that light from 20 ft or more will focus on your retina when the muscles are relaxed, so there is no effort in seeing. In your case, light from 20 ft focuses behind the retina, thus it is spread out when crossing the retina. We call this **far-sightedness**, because when you are young you can change focus using the lens inside the eye to focus the image onto the retina.

Usually, you do not notice problems far away, but you do up close, because then these muscles have to focus an extra amount. When using a computer 8 hours per day, these muscles are in continuous use; they weren't made for this. That is why your eyes tire by 1 o'clock in the afternoon. Also the muscles tend to "cramp up," causing the distance to blur at the end of the day. Now, whenever we change focus with these muscles, nervous energy is automatically sent to the outside muscles of the eye, causing them to turn inwards toward the target. In some cases, people's eyes turn in too much, in others they don't come in enough, like yours. That means you must compensate using another nervous system to the eyes. You don't do that very well, contributing to your tired eyes.

This is a picture of the back of your eye, with the nerve going to your brain and blood vessels coming into the eye. In diabetes, we can get new abnormal blood vessels growing that can cause a severe loss of vision. You don't show any hemorrhages or other indications of diabetes problems in the back of your eye, but we'll monitor that for you. When sugar levels are elevated, diabetes can also cause the lens in your eye to swell and cause you to become nearsighted, as well as contribute to dry eyes. Carefully check your glucose levels and listen to your internist concerning diet and exercise. I don't believe this is affecting your focusing or dry eyes at this time, but we'll watch for it.

Underneath your eyelids are hundreds of glands. You show hundreds of bumps. That is an allergic reaction to something like pollen. The glands do not secrete their tears, causing the eye to get dry and develop a burning sensation. Then your crying glands up here may flood the eyes with tears. They dry up and you go back through the cycle—dry, burn, flood. Normally, we blink 16–20 times a minute. When using a computer, this often drops to 5–7 times a minute, causing the eyes to dry out. I'm going to give you drops for the allergy condition and artificial tears to use during the day. We'll see if that takes care of the dry eye."

> In our example, Dr. Gates may finish his case presentation by say-
> ing, "In summary, I'm prescribing non-glare lenses for you to use at
> the computer, eye exercises to correct the muscle problem, and
> drops to improve the dry eye. I'll see you in 3 weeks and evaluate
> how you are responding to the treatment. Meanwhile, look over
> these suggestions for improving your workstation and watch your
> glucose levels."

In summary, doctors commonly use routing slips to indicate the prescribed treatment to staff, examination summaries, or additional testing, as explained in the computer vision evaluation form mentioned earlier in the chapter. Proper examination room decorating, use of carefully worded scripts by the doctor, and availability of patient education materials to reinforce the doctor's prescribed treatment will position the practice as the premier site for computer vision care.

Positioning the Practice in the Dispensary

The dispensary is the ideal location to demonstrate products available to treat CVS. It is often helpful if the dispensary can be seen from the reception area. Patients waiting for the doctor may hear happy, satisfied patients receiving their new computer eyewear. They can witness how the optician empathizes with the patients and relates to them. The dispensary can properly position your practice to the computer user through appearance, scripts for the optician, demonstrators, and patient education materials.

Dispensary Appearance

In addition to the décor options used for the reception room, pretesting room, and examination room, the dispensary should also have dispensing mats with computer vision themes as well as demonstrators, such as antireflective-coating demonstrators and lenses designed for computer users. PRIO is an optical company that provides colorful displays for their computer lenses and frames. You can review their products at http://www.prio.com.

Optician Scripts

We do not question the carefully chosen words that appear during a television commercial or movie, yet often we do not attend to how well we communicate in the office. Our computer-user patients are deciding on whether or not to spend a substantial amount of money to gain the benefits presented during the examination. Words chosen by the optician can reinforce those benefits or dismiss them. Phrases should be developed that reinforce the patient's decision to purchase computer glasses.

"I use the same lens design when I'm on my computer and it allows me to concentrate much better after a long day at the office!" Personal testimonials by the optician can be very effective. "The cost of computer glasses can be minimal when compared to the cost of other items we buy. Think about the cost per hour of that dress you are wearing? You will be wearing your computer glasses 8 hours a day, 5 days a week for 1 or 2 years! And that dress won't do anything for the comfort of your eyes at work!"

Allow your optician to develop scripts that are effective and give him or her some guidance as to what you believe complements what you are telling the patient.

Patient Education Materials

Most lens manufacturers provide brochures highlighting the advantages of their computer vision lenses. If none were given before this point in the visit, professional association pamphlets on computer vision may reinforce what the optician demonstrates to the patient. Some people use a "Computer Lens" information sheet like Figure 2-9. Hand these to the patient and tell him or her if any of his or her coworkers, friends, and family have any questions to give you a call. Remember, word of mouth is the best promoter of healthcare providers; the patients have the mouths, it is up to you to put the words in them.

COMPUTER GLASSES

More than 100 million Americans use computers every day at work. Seventy percent of them have vision problems. Using a computer presents a great demand on our eyes. The doctor has completed an examination designed to reveal problems that can limit your performance when using a computer. He has determined that you can benefit from wearing glasses designed specifically for computer use.

Focused for the computer. Glasses designed for the computer have many special features. The prescription will focus your eyes to allow minimal effort when trying to see at computer distances. Focusing your eyes for the computer allows the muscles inside your eye to relax, reducing the possibility of eyestrain and fatigue.

Non-glare lenses. The lenses prescribed for you are non-glare lenses. Glare is a constant cause of visual disturbance when using computers. Reflections off the surfaces of your spectacle lenses can result in loss of nearly 10% of light. This loss of light entering your eye decreases the contrast of the figures and letters. Loss of contrast can especially be a problem with those who have developing cataracts or macular degeneration. Reflections from the back of the spectacle lenses can also enter directly into the eye, causing irritating glare and degradation of the optical images. This glare is particularly noticeable in very nearsighted (myopic) individuals. The non-glare lens allows more light to the retina and reduces these reflections.

High-tech lens material. Today's technology allows lenses to be made from many different materials. Your lenses are composed of polycarbonate, the same material used in the aerospace industry and for compact disks. The benefit of this material is that it is nearly unbreakable. Polycarbonate is the safest lens material and is known as the most breakproof lens fabricated. The lens comes with a high-tech scratch-resistant coating, which allows it to last longer than other lenses.

Thin and light. Besides being breakage-resistant, your lenses are also the thinnest and lightest available. This lower weight allows your glasses to maintain the proper adjustment so all measurements remain in the correct place, allowing you the most usable vision.

High-tech lens design. The doctor prescribed the lens design that allows you the most use of your vision while using the computer. The design may take several forms. New technology has provided for designs specific to computer users. The new high-tech designs allow for normal head postures, which relax the neck and shoulder muscles. Musculoskeletal symptoms are often the result of improper head postures caused by poor lens design or measurements. The computer glasses manufactured for you are designed to give you maximal vision and maximal comfort.

*These glasses have been custom fit to your particular needs. There is probably no one else who can get the same benefits from them as you. As your eyes change in the future, we will alter your computer glasses to ensure you have comfort and maximize your performance. If you have any questions, please feel free to give us a call. Remember, our theme and our mission is to "**Provide you with good vision for the rest of your life!**" We have dedicated our lives to this purpose.*

FIGURE 2-9. Computer vision glasses patient handout.

Positioning the Practice at Checkout at the Front Desk

One of the responsibilities of the checkout person is to reinforce to patients that they made the right decision to invest in eyewear or services. If the front-desk person is using a computer, it is helpful for him or her to be wearing eyewear and to point out to the patients how happy they will be when they get their new computer glasses. A quick glance at the record can allow the receptionist to mention how the new glasses will solve the patient's problem of headaches, eye fatigue, or near blur (whatever was the chief entering complaint).

Another responsibility of the checkout staff is to reemphasize that the office is there to take care of all the patient's future vision needs.

"I know computers can be tough on your eyes. With today's technology, we can keep you comfortable at work and play and protect your vision into your old age. We'll give you a call in 1 year to set up your annual examination and let you know what new technologies have been developed that can benefit you. During the year, if anything comes up, don't hesitate to give us a call. As our office theme says, we are here to maintain your vision for the rest of your life!"

Positioning the Practice through Follow-Up

The time immediately after visiting your practice can be just as critical as during the examination visit. It is during this time that the patient questions whether the time and money spent in your office was worthwhile or not. Buyer's remorse is a common reaction for many of us, especially senior citizens. That is why it is so important that your staff reinforce the purchase decision at checkout and when picking up eyewear or receiving more services.

Follow-up is also critical to the referral of new patients. Sometimes patients are too overwhelmed with information to enable them to recall the "words" necessary for word-of-mouth promotion. Follow-up can give them the "words." Follow-up can be in the form of a phone call:

"I'm calling to learn how well those new glasses I prescribed for you have taken care of your headaches."

Rarely do doctors call to see how their patients are doing. This simple act can set you apart as special and caring. Patients are quick to tell their friends, who then question the caring attitudes of their own doctors. For computer users, the best follow-up would be an e-mail to see how they are doing. Complex cases requiring several treatment choices will result in a follow-up visit. Announcements, bulletins, and newsletters can easily be sent via e-mail to keep in touch with the computer-user patient.

Typical Computer-User Patient Flow with Performance Standards

Many offices create a checklist of activities expected during a patient visit to ensure that everyone is working together and supporting each other. Table 2-1 shows a sample computer-user patient flow checklist. From time to time, the list can accompany the patient file to document that each activity was completed. The purpose is to include all the service qualities stated by RATER at the beginning of this chapter. Paying attention to the little things that our computer-user patients value creates the proper atmosphere to encourage loyal, enthusiastic patients who refer coworkers, friends, and family.

The following chapters provide you with the tools necessary to diagnose and treat computer-related conditions.

Action Items

1. Consider how you can position your practice to computer users by designing the practice to be computer-user friendly: Where do you need to improve?
   • Before the patient visit
   • In the reception area

Table 2-1. Checklist for computer-user patient flow

Initial telephone call to make appointment
- ❏ Patient is asked when making appointment about computer usage by Virginia; notes that in file.
- ❏ Explains special concern office has for computer users.
- ❏ Smiles when speaking on phone.
- ❏ Encourages patient to check on office Web site.
- ❏ Says looking forward to meeting patient.

Entering office
- ❏ Enters practice and is greeted by Virginia using patient's name. "You must be Mrs. Gates? Welcome to Woodcrest Vision Center!"
- ❏ Tells patient about the office and doctor.
- ❏ Hands the patient a Welcome to the Office info packet.
- ❏ Watches to see if patient reads it.
- ❏ Offers a cold or hot drink and cookies.
- ❏ After patient peruses the info packet, Virginia brings a history form to her to fill out.
- ❏ Offers assistance and explains reason for history form to be filled out.

Pretesting room
- ❏ When the technician is ready, Virginia seats the patient in the pretesting room saying, "You'll like Julie. She explains things well and knows all about eyes and computers."
- ❏ Julie greets patient.
- ❏ Comments on competence of Virginia.
- ❏ Notes the computer usage on the history form and tells her about new products and services available to assist her visual comfort when on the computer.
- ❏ Gives her a computer-user–specific history form if appropriate.
- ❏ Begins pretesting, explaining every test and relating it to computer use.
- ❏ Hands patient brochures or pamphlets concerning computer vision.

Examination room
- ❏ Seats patient in examination room and tells her, "You'll like Dr. MacIntosh, he explains everything thoroughly, has 25 years' experience here in Woodcrest, and specializes in treating computer-user patients. Ask him about the computer lenses we discussed."
- ❏ Dr. MacIntosh greets patient.
- ❏ Comments on competence of Julie.
- ❏ Reviews history with patient and presents hypothesis as to cause.
- ❏ Conducts examination, explaining value of procedures and relating to probable treatment choice.
- ❏ Presents case to the patient and prescribed treatments.
- ❏ Completes summary form and hands to patient.
- ❏ Transfers patient to optician, "You'll like Marta, she will demonstrate the treatment I've prescribed for you and get you all set up! I'll see you again for a progress check on _____ to determine if there is anything else we must do for you."

Table 2-1. *Continued*

❑ Says goodbye.
Dispensary
❑ Marta comments on how competent and caring the doctor is.
❑ She reviews the treatment plan with the patient and demonstrates prescribed treatment as appropriate.
❑ Completes measurements and reviews costs, explaining benefits.
❑ Reinforces patient decision to purchase products.
❑ Says goodbye to patient.
Checkout at front desk
❑ Returns patient to Virginia at front desk to receive fees.
❑ Virginia comments on the competence and caring of Marta.
❑ She reinforces correctness of purchase decision.
❑ Schedules next appointment.
❑ Says goodbye to patient.
Follow-up
❑ Optician reinforces purchase decision at dispensing.
❑ Doctor or staff calls or e-mails patient to see how he or she is progressing.
❑ Follow-up appointment or additional treatment scheduled.
❑ E-mails sent to patient concerning computers and vision.
❑ Recall date set.

- With office forms
- In the pretesting room
- In the examination room
- In the dispensary
- Checking out at the front desk
- With follow-up

2. Develop a patient flow regimen to use with computer-user patients.

References

Moss GL, Shaw-McMinn PG. Eye Care Business: Marketing and Strategy. Boston: Butterworth–Heinemann, 2001.

3M Optical Systems Division. http://www.3M.com/cws. Accessed on May 2, 2002. 1-800-553-9215.

Parasuraman A, Berry L, Zeithami V. Understanding customer expectations of service. Sloan Management Review, Spring 1991;39–48.

Shaw-McMinn PG. CVS: The practical and the clinical. Rev Optom 2001;15:78–88.

Zeithami V, Parasuraman A, Berry L. Delivering Quality Service: Balancing Customer Perceptions and Expectations. New York: Free Press, 1990.

3
Signs and Symptoms of Computer Vision Problems

Eye and visual symptoms occur whenever the visual demands of the work exceed the individual's abilities to comfortably and efficiently deal with them. For example, gas station attendants do not complain of eyestrain. The visual demands of the tasks are simply not great enough to cause symptoms of eyestrain.

By comparison, many tasks, such as working at a computer (especially if the environmental conditions are poor), can cause symptoms in many working people because the visual demands exceed the capabilities of many of the workers. Eye-related symptoms occur in 25–93% of computer users, as reported by various investigators (Thompson, 1998). It is clear that a large percentage of computer workers experience eye symptoms. The large range is easily understood given the considerable variability in the methods of measuring symptoms, the wide range of jobs under study, and differences in eye care availability. Older workers and worker groups with poorer eye care, poorer computer displays, and poorer office ergonomics have more eye problems. There can be large prevalence differences among individual companies and even among different departments within the same company. Computer workers also experience musculoskeletal problems such as neck, back, shoulder, and wrist aches. A study by Hales and colleagues (1994) showed that 22% of computer workers have musculoskeletal disorders. Most studies show that eye-related problems are the most frequent health-related symptoms of computer workers.

Symptoms related to work almost always occur within a certain time period after the patient starts work. They are also dose related (Gunnarsson and Soderberg, 1983)—that is, the more intense the work, the more intense the symptoms. Normally, work-related symptoms go away on weekends and vacations. If the symptoms do not follow these patterns, they are probably not related to work.

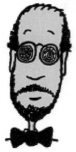
The presenting symptoms can be very helpful in identifying the most likely diagnosis—whether it is a visual or environmental diagnosis. A good case history directed toward exploring the patients' symptoms can often direct the examination and efficiently arrive at the diagnosis. This chapter focuses on the presenting symptoms of patients with computer vision syndrome. History forms and questions are provided to assist the assistant or technician in responding properly to the patient's concerns. This chapter also reviews the possible causes of the symptoms and how symptom analysis can efficiently direct the examination to the diagnosis. The chapter also describes how to prepare the patient for possible treatments before the examination begins.

Symptom Analysis

The symptoms that a particular computer worker has can be very helpful in identifying the most likely problem—whether the causative condition is visual, environmental, or both. Patient symptoms are most efficiently identified with a questionnaire designed for computer users. The questionnaire in Appendix 3-1 (page 44) is designed to identify the most important history information on a computer user. The categories of symptoms on the questionnaire are coordinated with the symptom categories discussed below.

Vision Symptoms

Blurred vision is a commonly reported symptom that usually points to a particular visual disorder (Box 3-1). Of course, constant blurred vision is an indication of an uncorrected refractive error or presbyopia, depending on the viewing distance at which the blur occurs. Squinting is also usually an indication of refractive error problems. Intermittent blurred vision at distance after near work is almost pathognomonic of an accommodative spasm or general accommoda-

> **Box 3-1**
>
> Visual symptoms
> - Blurred vision
> - Slow refocusing
> - Frequently losing place
> - Doubling of vision
> - Squinting
> - Changes in color perception

tive dysfunction. This blurred vision may only be momentary when the person looks up from his or her work or it can last for several hours after near work, causing difficulties driving home from work. If the blurred vision is intermittent at near viewing distances (slow refocusing) during near work, it almost certainly indicates an accommodative disorder such as reduced amplitude of accommodation or accommodative infacility. Testing should include amplitude of accommodation, lens flippers, and plus/minus lenses to blur binocularly (negative relative accommodation and positive relative accommodation). Sometimes a concurrent esophoria may be diagnosed as contributing to the accommodative problems.

Another cause of intermittent blurred vision at near viewing distances is dry eye. This can usually be differentiated in the history by asking the patient whether his or her vision clears when he or she blinks.

Diplopia (double vision) almost always indicates a binocular vision disorder, but careful questioning of patients or users is necessary to ensure that they are not reporting blurred vision as double vision. Intermittent diplopia that occurs after extended near work, especially if accompanied by reports of eyestrain, often indicates a convergence insufficiency. Repeated measurement of the near point of convergence should be performed and ability to comfortably maintain fixation at the near point of convergence should be evaluated.

However, patients seldom report diplopia, even if their eyes become momentarily misaligned. People are so intolerant of seeing

Box 3-2

Ocular symptoms
- Irritated eyes
- Itching and burning eyes
- Excessive tears
- Dry eyes
- Excessive blinking
- Contact lens discomfort
- Sore or hurting eyes

double that as soon as it happens they close their eyes or in some other manner quickly discontinue the viewing situation that results in double vision. The lack of diplopia as a symptom does not in any way rule out the possibility of a binocular vision disorder.

Color perception problems were more frequent with older monochrome video display terminals; however, they can still occur in situations in which the user spends considerable time viewing a saturated color. This problem is managed by changing to less saturated and dimmer colors on the computer display. See Chapter 10 for further information on this topic.

Ocular Symptoms

In computer workers, any of the symptoms listed in Box 3-2 typically indicate dry eyes (see Chapter 7). Computer workers are particularly prone to having dry eye problems because their blink rate is significantly reduced and their horizontal gaze angle at the screen results in an ocular aperture which is larger than when looking down and reading a book, thereby resulting in increased tear evaporation. A report of watery eyes is often the result of reflex tearing secondary to irritation caused by dry eyes. Tear film quality and tear quantity should be investigated. Many patients with marginal dry eyes have no symptoms during other daily activities, but have significant dry eye symptoms when working at the computer.

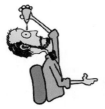

If a patient reports symptoms of dry eyes, ask whether the computer screen is too high (the center of the screen should be 4–9 in. below the eyes), whether the office is low in humidity (particularly a problem during cold weather), or if he or she is seated with a vent aimed toward his or her eyes. Affirmative answers to these questions identify environmental problems that can be important in resolving the patient's symptoms.

Itching eyes often indicate seasonal allergy problems and should be pursued with further questions. Also, irritated or burning eyes in the absence of dry eye findings may indicate airborne toxicants in the office environment. This is further indicated if other employees in the work area have similar symptoms.

Asthenopic Symptoms

The group of symptoms listed in Box 3-3 includes eyestrain, headaches, and eye fatigue. This set of symptoms is the least diagnostic group of symptoms; there are numerous diagnostic conditions that can cause these symptoms. These conditions include uncorrected refractive error, presbyopia, accommodative disorders, esophoria, convergence insufficiency, and poor ergonomics such as glare from overhead lights.

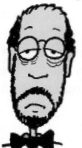

A report of eye or general fatigue associated with near work can often indicate a convergence insufficiency. If the patient is exophoric, carefully evaluate the base-out to blur findings and the near point of convergence. If the patient is noticeably strained during near point of convergence testing, ask whether he or she feels the same strain when working. Very often, the patient will report that the strain is identical, thereby confirming the diagnosis in both the doctor's and the patient's mind. This facilitates patient motivation for the most effective treatment—convergence training.

It is unfortunate that a patient report of eyestrain does not provide a strong clue to any diagnosis, because eyestrain is the most commonly reported symptom by patients working at computers. Additional questioning can often elicit more specific descriptions of the symptoms.

> **Box 3-3**
>
> General eye symptoms—asthenopia
> - Eyestrain
> - Headache
> - Eye fatigue
> - Tired eyes

Light Sensitivity Symptoms

Many patients report sensitivity to lights (especially fluorescent lights) or that flickering light bothers them (Box 3-4). Iritis can cause these symptoms and should be ruled out.

The most common cause of light sensitivity problems among computer users is lighting in the work environment. It is common for computer workers to experience discomfort glare from overhead fluorescent lights or from bright windows. This is due to the fact that computer workers have a higher gaze angle in the room compared to other desk workers, resulting in the bright lights being closer to central fixation. This condition can be diagnosed by having the patient shield his or her eyes from offending light sources. An immediate sense of relief indicates that the patient is experiencing glare discomfort, and he or she should either eliminate the glare source or wear a visor. Glare discomfort can be demonstrated in the office (in a location with bright overhead lights) so that the patient knows what to look for back at his or her own desk. Decreasing the brightness of the computer screen

> **Box 3-4**
>
> Lighting symptoms
> - Flickering sensations
> - Glare
> - Light sensitivity

(thereby decreasing sensitivity to flicker) or prescribing a pink tint lens can also help alleviate the symptoms of light sensitivity.

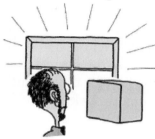

Some patients report flicker of the computer display. This is possible if the patient uses a cathode ray tube (instead of a liquid crystal display) and the refresh rate is relatively low—say 60–70 Hz. These symptoms can often be eliminated by adjusting the refresh rate higher, decreasing the display brightness, or both. See Chapter 10.

In some situations, a binocular vision disorder can result in light sensitivity. Light sensitivity occurs because it is difficult to suppress an image in brighter light. This failure to suppress causes symptoms from the attempt to gain and maintain binocularity. The difficulty of suppressing in bright light is why an intermittent strabismic squints in the sun but not indoors. The squinter often has no idea he or she is closing one eye. Visual therapy improves the ability to compensate and fuse, thereby eliminating the need to suppress to avoid binocular problems.

Musculoskeletal Symptoms

Many patients who maintain the same posture for extended periods of time report neck aches, shoulder aches, or backaches. This is common for many computer workers as well as for microscopists, assembly line workers, and others engaged in repetitive work. These musculoskeletal symptoms result from assuming a less than optimal posture for extended periods of time, which causes tonic stress in the musculature (Box 3-5).

Box 3-5

Musculoskeletal symptoms
- Neck or shoulder tension, pain
- Back pain
- Pain in arms, wrists, or shoulders

These problems are often related to the eyes. It is commonly recognized that "the eyes lead the body." For visually intensive tasks, the body locates the eyes at a position where they can comfortably and efficiently perform the job; this is often accomplished by creating awkward posture that results in musculoskeletal problems.

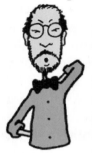 If multifocal lenses do not provide the correct lens power at the correct location in the lens for the patient's work, they cause the person to assume an awkward position and thus cause musculoskeletal symptoms. It is important to know the viewing distances and locations of the patient's work (see the questionnaire in Appendix 3-1, page 44) so that the proper prescription and lens design can be made. It can be very helpful to have patients bring measurements of their work location with them to the examination, but it is often easier to have patients go back to their work area and return with the critical measurements.

If the patient's workstation is not properly set up for him or her, it can easily result in these musculoskeletal symptoms. For example, if the patient's computer screen is too high or off to the side it can result in neck aches, backaches, or both. Shoulder aches are often caused by keyboards that are too high.

Box 3-6

General symptoms

- Tension
- Excessive physical fatigue
- Irritability
- Increased nervousness
- More frequent errors
- General fatigue, drowsiness

Other Symptoms

Many computer workers have stressful jobs, often compounded by personal problems. Symptoms of tension, irritability, and others are common and usually are not related to eye problems. However, it is not uncommon for eye-related problems to work in synergy with other life and work stressors to produce these general symptoms (Box 3-6).

References

Gunnarsson E, Soderberg I. Eye strain resulting from VDU work at the Swedish Telecommunications Administration. Appl Ergon 1983;14:61–69.

Hales TR, Sauter SL, Peterson MR, et al. Musculoskeletal disorders among visual display terminal users in a telecommunications company. Ergonomics 1994;37:1603–1621.

Thompson WD. Eye problems and visual display terminals—the facts and fallacies. Ophthalmic Physiol Opt 1998;18(2):111–119.

Appendix 3-1

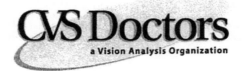

Dear Patient,
Please take a few moments to fill out this questionnaire and bring it with you to the examination. In this way we can best resolve the problems you may be having at your computer.

Identify the symptoms you experience. Also, comment about the severity and frequency of occurrence.

Visual
_____ Blurred vision
_____ Slow refocusing
_____ Frequently losing place
_____ Doubling of vision
_____ Squinting
_____ Changes in color perception

Ocular
_____ Irritated eyes
_____ Itching and burning eyes
_____ Excessive tears
_____ Dry eyes
_____ Excessive blinking
_____ Contact lens discomfort
_____ Sore or hurting eyes

General—eye
_____ Eyestrain
_____ Headache
_____ Eye fatigue
_____ Tired eyes

Light

_____ Flickering sensations

_____ Glare

_____ Light sensitivity

Muscle

_____ Neck or shoulder tension, pain

_____ Back pain

_____ Pain in arms, wrists, or shoulders

Other

_____ Tension

_____ Excessive physical fatigue

_____ Irritability

_____ Increased nervousness

_____ More frequent errors

_____ General fatigue, drowsiness

How many hours per day do you work at the computer? _____

How long before the symptoms occur? _____

Do your symptoms persist even when you are not working? **Yes No**
   If YES, please describe:

Are your eyes **higher** or **lower** (circle one) than the center of the computer screen?

_____ By how much?

_____ Distance from eyes to center of computer screen with usual posture

_____ Distance from eyes to reference documents

Y N Are there bright lights (e.g., windows or overhead lights) in your field of view while looking at the computer?

Y N If so, does shielding your eyes from the bright lights make you feel more comfortable?

Y N Does shielding the screen (e.g., with a file folder) from overhead lights or bright windows improve the screen visibility?

4
Diagnosis and Treatment of Refractive Errors for Computer Users

An uncorrected refractive error can result in some of the symptoms that computer workers experience.

The condition of myopia, by itself, does not usually cause symptoms for a computer user. In fact, many myopes can use their eyes more comfortably at near working distances by taking their glasses off. Without glasses, the myope can see near objects without using as much accommodation as a person with emmetropia. (With glasses on, the myope uses approximately the same amount of accommodation as an emmetrope.) Because the extended use of accommodation can cause symptoms, as is discussed more fully in Chapter 5, the myope can be at a comfort advantage without glasses on.

Myopes with low to moderate amounts of myopia can often read comfortably without their glasses at normal viewing distances. For example, a –2.50 diopter (D) myope can read at 40 cm (16 in.) without using accommodation, a 3.00 D myope at 33 cm (13 in.). (A 10.00 D myope is great at inspecting jewelry at 4 in. without glasses on!)

There is one problem, however, that a low to moderate myope can experience at a computer. The person with 2.00–3.00 D of myopia who is used to taking his or her glasses off for normal reading is unable to see the computer screen clearly with his or her glasses off because it is located farther away than the usual reading distance. The patient may need to assume an awkward posture to obtain a shorter distance to the computer screen. Wearing the distance glasses may enable the patient to see the screen clearly, but sometimes he or she cannot comfortably use his or her accommodation through the glasses.

Myopia Development

It is generally accepted, and most studies support the concept, that there is a strong genetic factor in the development of myopia (Edwards and Lewis, 1991; Teikari et al., 1991; Krause et al., 1993; Yap et al., 1993; Zadnik et al., 1994). A 24-year longitudinal study showed that children with two myopic parents are 6.42 times as likely to develop myopia compared to children with one or no myopic parents (Pacella et al., 1999). The genetic input to myopia development is strong; the more relevant issue concerning work at computer displays is whether the manner in which a person uses his or her eyes has an influence on the development of myopia.

Many studies have indicated that working at near distances can result in the development of some myopia. The introduction of school systems to cultures in which they did not previously exist has resulted in a greater incidence of myopia (Young et al., 1970), presumably because of increased near work. Individuals who do a tour of duty on a submarine (Kinney et al., 1980), in which all viewing distances are restricted, show increases in myopia. There is also a large percentage of microscopists who have myopia and who develop it in their adult years (Adams and McBrien, 1992). Monkeys raised in cages with restricted viewing distances also have been shown to develop myopia (Young, 1961, 1981). Sperduto et al. (1983) measured a positive association between myopia and both income level and near work in the population. Several cross-sectional studies have found associations between near work and myopia progression (Richler and Bear, 1980; Wong et al., 1993; Zylbermann et al., 1993; Saw et al., 1996; Saw et al., 1999). Saw et al. (2000), however, studied myopia progression in 153 Singaporean children and determined higher progression rates for younger children and those with higher amounts of myopia at the beginning of the study, but no correlation was measured with the amount of near work. Tan et al. (2000) likewise found no correlation between the amount of near work and myopia progression in a group of 168 Singaporean children; however, they measured significantly higher rates of progression immediately after the children took examinations. The preponderance of these studies supports the contention that near work is associated with myopia development in some people.

Accommodation may play a role in myopia development. The use of atropine on monkeys, which paralyzes accommodation, results in no myopia development. Accommodation is further implicated in the myopia development process by the finding that bifocals for children, which negate the need for accommodation, lessen the development of myopia compared to a control group (Oakley and Young, 1975). These results have been verified in some, but not all, studies into the effectiveness of bifocals or progressive addition lenses at decreasing the progression of myopia (Goss and Grosvenor, 1990; Goss, 1994; Leung and Brown, 1999; Ong et al., 1999). In particular, Leung and Brown determined a statistically significant lower amount of myopia progression in a test group of 36 children who wore progressive addition lenses compared to a control group of 32 children who wore single vision lenses. Subjects in both groups were selected to have a record of recent myopia progression of at least –0.40 D per year. Test group subjects were prescribed +1.50 or +2.00 D add. Those with +2.00 add showed less myopia progression than those wearing +1.50 add. The clinical use of a near lens addition seems effective at reducing myopia progression.

Numerous laboratory studies on animals have shown the strong influence that visual stimulation during development can have on adult refractive error (reviewed by Norton and Siegwart, 1995). A generally accepted physiologic model has developed that supports the effects of environment on end-state refractive error. Animal experiments on chickens (Irving et al., 1992; Wallman et al., 1995; Wildsoet and Wallman, 1995), tree shrews (Siegwart and Norton, 1993), and monkeys (Hung et al., 1995) have shown that axial length changes during eye development compensate the defocus created by wearing spectacle lenses. This has been shown to be a very robust effect. The evidence supports the concept that blur on the retina stimulates axial length growth of the eye, and that such growth terminates when a clear image is obtained at the retina. Such a mechanism would also explain the fact that emmetropia is much more common in the population than would be expected on the basis of normal distribution. These animal studies support the contention that work at near distances can result in an environmentally determined myopia.

It has been shown that esophoria is a risk factor for myopia development in children (Goss, 1990, 1991; Goss and Jackson, 1996). This finding is interesting theoretically and clinically. Esophoria often results in a larger accommodative lag, resulting in retinal blur (Goss and Rainey, 1999). If, as in the animal model, blur is a stimulus for axial length growth in humans, then the retinal blur created by esophoria could be a causative factor in the myopia that is associated with esophoria. From a clinical management point of view, this suggests that myopia development may be more likely to be associated with near work if the patient has an esophoria at near. Another caution in applying these findings is that the association between esophoria and myopia development has been established for pediatric populations, not adults.

The findings reported so far provide compelling evidence that near work is associated with the development of myopia in some people. However, does this apply to viewing a computer display? Or is the effect any different for viewing computer displays compared to viewing other near objects?

Tokoro (1988) reported myopic progression in 437 subjects after 1 year of an unspecified amount of work at computers. No control group of adults performing other forms of near work was used, so the results cannot apply specifically to viewing computer displays. Toppel and Neuber (1994) studied refractive error change over 2 years in 107 computer workers compared to a control group of 69 persons who never used a computer. Likewise, Boos et al. (1985) studied refractive error changes in 505 computer workers compared to 126 non-computer workers. Both of these controlled studies measured no difference in myopia progression between the computer-using and control groups. Yeow and Taylor (1991) matched 32 pairs of female computer users and non-users for age and initial refractive error. They measured no difference in refractive error change between the groups. Mutti and Zadnik (1996) have identified numerous challenges in properly designing a study to definitively test whether viewing a computer display causes higher risk of myopia development compared to other types of work. However, given the limitations of previous studies and their assessment of the literature, Mutti and Zadnik (1996) concluded that there is no compelling evidence to believe that work at a computer display creates significant risk for myopia development compared to other forms of near work.

Considerable evidence supports the contention that extended near work is a risk factor for myopia development—whether the near work involves viewing a computer display or other near objects. There is no evidence, however, to indicate that working at a computer display creates any greater risk for myopia than other forms of near work.

Transient changes in myopia are common after work at a computer and other forms of near work. Yeow and Taylor (1989) showed a myopic shift on average of –0.12 D in a group of computer workers, whereas no shift occurred in a control group of non-computer workers. Transient myopia was also reported by Watten and Lie (1992). However, Rosenfield and Ciuffreda (1994) have shown that transient myopia can occur simply by viewing a printed page at 20 cm for 10 minutes. Transient myopic changes have been shown objectively to result from temporary changes in accommodation (Ciuffreda and Ordonez, 1995). Further discussion about the literature and the clinical diagnosis and management of this condition is in Chapter 5.

The preponderance of the evidence supports the idea that near work, in some way, places a person at greater risk for the development of myopia. This is particularly true for children (Goss, 1994). Clearly, this does not happen to everyone; otherwise, every school child and every near-point worker would develop myopia.

Based on clinical experience, it is common for some young adults, usually aged 20–30 years, to develop a late-onset myopia that has coincided with beginning intensive near work and, in many cases, using a computer. The amount of this late-onset myopia is usually 1.00 D or less. Although this late-onset myopia occurs among computer workers, it also occurs among college students, accountants, book-keepers, and others who work for extended periods of time at near working distances. There is no evidence to implicate work at a computer display as causing myopia any more than other forms of extended near work. Viewing a computer display is not the specific culprit for the myopia that develops, but rather near work more generally. Environmentally determined myopia is still not well understood; it is possible that future study may provide information to better determine what aspect or aspects of near work are responsible for the myopia development.

Many individuals who develop late-onset myopia also have an accommodative disorder or a binocular vision disorder at near working distances. Research suggests that esophoria at near results in a greater chance of myopia development. The primary complaint of patients with late-onset myopia is distance blur. Of course, a distance refractive correction is the best management of this problem. Some patients are concerned about etiology of the myopia and interested in possible remedy. Regression of the myopia with treatment is unusual; however, favorable findings include esophoria at near, an accommodative disorder, significant reduction in myopia with cycloplegia, or a combination of these. If the myopia development is caught early and treatment of the near visual disorder is instituted, the myopia development may regress or stabilize. The near visual treatment consists of reading glasses or vision training.

Hyperopia

A person with hyperopia and an adequate amount of accommodation can use accommodative effort to add refractive power to the eye and, therefore, see distant objects clearly. However, without an adequate amount of accommodation, the hyperopic patient is unable to see distant objects clearly, or, if able to do so, only for short periods of time. This situation is even worse when viewing near objects. If the amount of hyperopia is low and the individual is young with a large amount of accommodation, then near objects might be able to be cleared comfortably. But, more often, the dual demands on accommodation of the hyperopia and the near viewing distance can exceed the accommodative abilities of the individual.

Hyperopia is most commonly corrected with spectacles or contact lenses that have positive refractive power. Although the condition of hyperopia may have existed in an individual since childhood, the onset of symptoms or poor vision caused by the hyperopia may not occur until adulthood. The first problems with hyperopia usually occur at near working distances. Hyperopia usually manifests as symptoms of eyestrain or headaches, or may manifest as intermittent blurring of near work.

Of course, because the ability to accommodate decreases with age (see Chapter 5), the ability to compensate for a hyperopia decreases with age. The age at which a given individual needs to first obtain a hyperopic correction depends on the dioptric value of the hyperopia, the state of the individual's accommodative system, and the amount of near work.

As is discussed in Chapter 5, work at a computer display can be particularly demanding on the accommodative mechanism. Therefore, many adults with low amounts of hyperopia need to have the hyperopia corrected for work at a computer, although they might not otherwise need the correction (at that time). Many patients with hyperopia of only 0.50–1.00 D have symptoms of eyestrain at near working distances, and correction of the hyperopia relieves the symptoms. They usually only need to wear the corrective glasses for near work. If these individuals were not performing a job that required extensive use of their eyes at near distances, they would not yet need the hyperopic correction. However, because work at a computer is demanding of near vision, they require the correction for comfortable vision.

Astigmatism

A significant astigmatism can create blur at all working distances. Wiggins and Daum (1991) and Wiggins et al. (1992) have shown that uncorrected astigmatic errors of 0.50 D are significantly associated with visual discomfort for work at computer displays. Astigmatism creates blur regardless of the viewing distance. Even small amounts of blur can cause decreased performance and visual discomfort. If the astigmatism is 0.50 D or greater, it should be considered as a potential problem and should be corrected.

Refractive Error—Clinical Care Summary

Many patients simply need an accurate correction of refractive error (myopia, hyperopia, or astigmatism) (Daum et al., 1988). The blur created by the refractive error makes it more difficult to easily acquire visual information. Astigmatism of 0.50 D or greater is associated with visual discomfort in clinical studies and should be considered for correction.

Patients with hyperopia must exert more accommodative effort than non-hyperopes to see clearly at near distances. Therefore, many hyperopic computer users require refractive correction, although they may not require it for a less visually demanding job. Hyperopia of 0.50 D or greater should be considered for prescription, in consideration of the age of the patient and his or her accommodative findings.

Patients with 2.00–3.50 D of myopia who habitually read without their glasses often have visual and musculoskeletal difficulties at the computer because the computer working distance is greater than that at which they usually read. They need to posture themselves too close to the computer to see clearly without their glasses. They may be able to use their distance glasses at the computer—assuming good accommodative function. However, these patients often have a subpar accommodative mechanism and therefore require a partial correction of their myopia for proper function at the computer display.

Some computer-using patients present with a recently developed myopia of 0.25–1.00 D, the onset of which closely coincides with beginning extended work on a computer or other near work. Some of these patients have an accommodative disorder or an esophoria at near working distance, correction of which may (or, most often, will not) retard or stop the progression of the myopia. Usually the refractive error at distance should be corrected, unless the uncorrected distance acuity is adequate for the distant visual needs of the patient. Table 4-1 summarizes the prescribing needs of refractive errors.

Visual Acuity

Good visual acuity is essential for performance and comfort when viewing a computer display. Research, as reviewed in Chapter 10, has shown that even small improvements in display quality result in significant improvements in comfort and reading performance. Also, as reviewed in Chapter 10, the visual acuity should be three times better than that required to read the text on the display (i.e.,

TABLE 4-1. Prescribing for distance refractive errors

Type of refractive error	Amount of distance refractive error	Comments
Hyperopia	>+0.50	Correct if there are symptoms—especially if concerned about accommodative function
Myopia	>−2.00	Correct partially for near vision *if* the patient removes glasses for near work
Myopia	Any	Correct for distance tasks as indicated
Astigmatism	>0.50	Correct in presence of symptoms

there should be a 3× acuity reserve). If a person has 20/25 acuity, then the text on the screen should be at least 20/75 in size for the viewing distance.

It is important to provide the patient with optimal visual acuity. However, to have optimal performance and comfort, the patient should be viewing text that meets the 3× rule. This is most frequently an issue with older patients with reduced acuity and contrast sensitivity. Any patient with reduced visual acuity or contrast sensitivity is at higher risk for having the screen characters appear too small. If you have concerns about text size for your patient, a method for testing the 3× rule is presented in Box 4-1.

Myopia and astigmatism certainly reduce visual acuity. Hyperopia reduces visual acuity less predictably because younger individuals can use their accommodative mechanism (eye-focusing ability) to add power to the eye to eliminate or reduce the blur caused by the hyperopia. Accommodative ability predictably declines with age (thus necessitating reading glasses or bifocals). Therefore, the visual acuity losses due to myopia and hyperopia approach one another as we look at progressively older age groups.

However, we cannot overlook that the primary reason for correcting refractive errors is to obtain an improvement in visual acuity. Given the fact that the size and clarity of letters presented on computer displays makes them difficult to see, it is wise to obtain a good visual acuity. Industrial screening programs should select 20/25 acuity

Box 4-1

Self-test for character size to meet the 3× rule

Clinician guidelines: For best viewing of the characters on the computer screen, first prescribe appropriately for the patient's optimal viewing distance, then have the patient move back to three times that distance, and determine whether he or she can still discriminate the characters. For presbyopic patients, variable focus design lenses are best for this self-test, because they focus at 4–6 ft in the top of the lenses; however, the distance prescription can usually be used for the 3× distance. If the computer user is unable to distinguish the characters on the screen, adjust the display size until they can just be discriminated at triple the normal computer-to-eye distance.

as the criterion for passing. Acuities poorer than this do not allow for enough acuity reserve. For a discussion of the relationship between visual acuity and letter size on the display, see Character Size and the 3× Rule in Chapter 10.

Summary

Proper correction of refractive error is essential to the eye care of most computer users. Because of the high visual demands of the task, even small refractive errors can cause blur and result in symptoms. This can be particularly true for low amounts of astigmatism, which result in blur or low amounts of hyperopia, which can result in blur and increased use of accommodation. Patients with low to moderate amounts of myopia who remove their glasses for near work may be at risk for postural problems because the computer display is farther away than most reading materials. Partial prescription for the myopia, or the equivalent of a near add, should be considered for such patients. Although there is some scientific basis to support extended near work causing the development of myopia in some people, there is no evidence to support the idea that viewing a computer display increases such risk. Chapter 5 explains the role of accommodation and binocularity in affecting the comfort of computer users.

Action Items

1. Decide how distance refractive error will impact the prescription you give to the prepresbyopic patient. Use the exercise in Appendix 4-1 (page 60) to practice.
2. Train your staff and develop a script on what you are going to say to the patient concerning the effect of computer work on the refractive status of his or her eyes.
3. Train your staff and compose a script on how to determine the optimum character size to provide maximal visual comfort.
4. Have staff develop an in-office demonstration of how to determine optimum character size.

References

Adams DW, McBrien NA. Prevalence of myopia and myopic progression in a population of clinical microscopists. Optom Vis Sci 1992;69(6):467–473.

Boos SR, Calissendorff BM, Knave BG. Work with video display terminals among office employees. III. Ophthalmological factors. Scand J Work Environ Health 1985;11(6):475–481.

Ciuffreda KJ, Ordonez X. Abnormal transient myopia in symptomatic individuals after sustained near work. Optom Vis Sci 1995;72(7):506–510.

Daum KM, Good G, Tijerina L. Symptoms in video display terminal operators and the presence of small refractive errors. J Am Optom Assoc 1988;59:691–697.

Edwards M, Lewis WH. Autosomal recessive inheritance of myopia in Hong Kong Chinese infants. Ophthalmic Physiol Opt 1991;11(3):227–231.

Goss DA. Variables related to the rate of childhood myopia progression. Optom Vis Sci 1990;67:631–636.

Goss DA. Clinical accommodation and heterophoria findings preceding juvenile onset of myopia. Optom Vis Sci 1991;68:110–116.

Goss DA. Effect of spectacle correction on the progression of myopia in children—a literature review. J Am Optom Assoc 1994;65(2):117–128.

Goss DA, Grosvenor T. Rates of childhood myopia progression with bifocals as a function of nearpoint phoria: consistency of three studies. Optom Vis Sci 1990;67(8):637–640.

Goss DA, Jackson T. Clinical findings before the onset of myopia in youth: 3. Heterophoria. Optom Vis Sci 1996;73:269–278.

Goss DA, Rainey B. Relationship of accommodative response and nearpoint phoria in a sample of myopic children. Optom Vis Sci 1999;76(5):292–294.

Hung LF, Crawford ML, Smith EL. Spectacle lenses alter eye growth and the refractive status of young monkeys. Nat Med 1995;1(8):761–765.

Irving EL, Sivak JG, Callendar MG. Refractive plasticity of the developing chick eye. Ophthalmic Physiol Opt 1992;12(4):448–456.

Kinney JAS, Luria SM, Ryan AP, et al. The vision of submariners and national guardsmen: a longitudinal study. Am J Optom Physiol Opt 1980;57:469–478.

Krause UH, Rantakallio PT, Koiranen MJ, Mottonen JK. The development of myopia up to the age of twenty and a comparison of refraction in parents and children. Arctic Med Res 1993;52(4):161–165.

Leung J, Brown B. Progression of myopia in Hong Kong Chinese schoolchildren is slowed by wearing progressive lenses. Optom Vis Sci 1999;76(6):346–354.

Mutti DO, Zadnik K. Is computer use a risk factor for myopia? J Am Optom Assoc 1996;67:521–530.

Norton TT, Siegwart JT. Animal models of emmetropization: matching axial length to the focal plane. J Am Optom Assoc 1995;66(7):405–414.

Oakley KH, Young FA. Bifocal control of myopia. Am J Optom Physiol Opt 1975; 52:758.

Ong E, Grice K, Held R, et al. Effects of spectacle intervention on the progression of myopia in children. Optom Vis Sci 1999;76(6):363–369.

Pacella R, McLellan J, Grice K, et al. Role of genetic factors in the etiology of juvenile-onset myopia based on a longitudinal study of refractive error. Optom Vis Sci 1999;76(6):381–386.

Richler A, Bear J. Refraction, near work and education. A population study in Newfoundland. Acta Ophthalmol (Copenh) 1980;58:468–478.

Rosenfield M, Ciuffreda KJ. Cognitive demand and transient near-work-induced myopia. Optom Vis Sci 1994;71(6):381–385.

Saw S, Chia S, Chew S. Relation between work and myopia in Singapore women. Optom Vis Sci 1999;76:393–396.

Saw S, Katz J, Schein O, et al. Epidemiology of myopia. Epidemiol Rev 1996;18:175–187.

Saw S, Nieto F, Katz J, et al. Factors related to the progression of myopia in Singaporean children. Optom Vis Sci 2000;77(10):549–554.

Siegwart JT, Norton TT. Refractive and ocular changes in tree shrews raised with plus or minus lenses. Invest Ophthalmol Vis Sci 1993;34(4):1208.

Sperduto RD, Seigel D, Roberts J, Rowland M. Prevalence of myopia in the United States. Arch Ophthalmol 1983;101:405–407.

Tan N, Saw S, Lam D, et al. Temporal variations in myopia progression in Singaporean children within an academic year. Optom Vis Sci 2000;77(9):465–472.

Teikari JM, O'Donnell J, Kaprio J, Koskenvuo M. Impact of heredity in myopia. Hum Hered 1991;41(3):151–156.

Tokoro T. Effect of visual display terminal (VDT) work on myopia progression. Acta Ophthalmol 1988;66(Suppl 185):172–174.

Toppel L, Neuber M. Evaluation of refractive values in patients working for several years at video display terminals. A long-term study. Ophthalmologe 1994;91(1): 103–106.

Wallman J, Wildsoet C, Xu A. Moving the retina: choroidal modulation of refractive state. Vision Res 1995;35(1):37–50.

Watten RG, Lie I. Time factors in VDT-induced myopia and visual fatigue: an experimental study. J Hum Ergol (Tokyo) 1992;21(1):13–20.

Wiggins NP, Daum KM. Visual discomfort and astigmatic refractive errors in VDT use. J Am Optom Assoc 1991;62(9):680–684.

Wiggins NP, Daum KM, Snyder CA. Effects of residual astigmatism in contact lens wear on visual discomfort in VDT use. J Am Optom Assoc 1992;63(3):177–181.

Wildsoet C, Wallman J. Choroidal and scleral mechanisms of compensation for spectacle lenses in chicks. Vision Res 1995;35(9):1175–1194.

Wong L, Coggon D, Cruddas M, Hwang C. Education, reading and familial tendency as risk factors for myopia in Hong Kong fisherman. J Epidemiol Community Health 1993;47:50–53.

Yap M, Wu M, Liu ZM, et al. Role of heredity in the genesis of myopia. Ophthalmic Physiol Opt 1993;13(3):316–319.

Yeow PT, Taylor SP. Effects of short-term VDT usage on visual functions. Optom Vis Sci 1989;66(7):459–466.

Yeow PT, Taylor SP. Effects of long-term visual display terminal usage on visual functions. Optom Vis Sci 1991;68(12):930–941.

Young FA. The development and retention of myopia by monkeys. Am J Optom Arch Am Acad Optom 1961;38(10):545–555.

Young FA. Primate myopia. Am J Optom Physiol Opt 1981;58(7):560–566.

Young FA, Leary GA, Baldwin WR, et al. Refractive errors, reading performance, and school achievement among Eskimo children. Am J Optom Arch Am Acad Optom 1970;47:384.

Zadnik K, Satariano WA, Mutti DO, et al. The effect of parental history of myopia on children's eye size. JAMA 1994;271(17):1323–1327.

Zylbermann R, Landau D, Berson D. The influence of study habits on myopia in Jewish teenagers. J Pediatr Ophthalmol Strabismus 1993;30:319–322.

Appendix 4-1

How would you manage the following prepresbyopic computer-using patients?

1. A 21 year old presenting with blurred distance vision. The patient is comfortable working at the computer for long hours. You find a refractive error of –0.50 sphere, 20/20 OU.
2. A 24 year old presenting with eyes tiring after 30 minutes of using the computer. You find a refractive error of +0.25 –0.50 × 90, 20/20 OU.
3. A 25 year old presenting with eyes tiring after using the computer for short periods of time. A cycloplegic refraction shows a distance refractive error of +0.50 sphere, 20/20 OU.
4. A 29 year old reporting that she prefers to use her computer without her habitual glasses, but she must get too close to the monitor to comfortably view it. Testing shows a distance refractive error equal to her present glasses of –2.75 sphere 20/20 OU.
5. A 24 year old enters presenting with distance blur. You measure –0.50 sphere OU. A previous examination 2 years earlier showed a refractive error of +0.25 OU. The patient asks if the computer caused the myopia. How do you respond?

5

Diagnosis and Treatment of Accommodative and Binocular Conditions

Viewing a computer display can be demanding on the accommodative mechanism. Accommodative ability, often as it interacts with refractive error, can affect the comfort of computer users and cause symptoms such as those listed in Box 5-1. This chapter provides a review of the accommodative and binocular responses to computer displays and discusses how to diagnose and treat accommodative and binocular disorders.

Accommodation

An improperly functioning accommodative mechanism is normally the cause of intermittent blurring of near objects, such as the computer screen or reference documents, and is also responsible for temporary blurring of distant objects after working at near distances. Intermittent blurring of near objects is caused by an inability of the accommodative mechanism to maintain a steady focus on near objects. Blurring of distant objects occurs when, after extended near work, the ciliary muscle remains fixed or somewhat locked in the near contracted position. This effectively makes the eye myopic when looking at distance. When the ciliary muscle functions properly, distant objects should become clear in less than half of a second after looking at a near object. Sometimes a worker notices that it takes a few seconds to clear a distant object, such as a clock on a wall, after looking up from the computer screen. Some-

> **Box 5-1**
>
> Symptoms associated with accommodative dysfunction
> - Near blur
> - Post-work distance blur
> - Asthenopia
> - Headache

times this distant blurring can last for several hours after extended near work, often affecting driving. An improperly functioning accommodative mechanism can also result in symptoms of eyestrain and headaches.

Patients with accommodative disorders can generally be treated with spectacles that relieve the accommodative effort required to see clearly at near working distances. Some accommodative disorders can also be treated with vision training exercises.

Amplitude of Accommodation and Effects of Age

One of the primary clinical measures of accommodation is the amplitude of accommodation. The amplitude is measured by locating the closest distance to the eye at which the person can still keep a clear focus on an object with small detail. The distance from the eye (usually the spectacle plane) is noted (in meters) and then converted to diopters (D) by taking the inverse.

There is a clear and well-known relationship between the amplitude of accommodation and age. Borish (1970) provides a good historical review of the research on age and amplitude of accommodation. Donders (1864) was the first to establish a relationship between the age of accommodation and the expected diopters of accommodation. He measured 130 subjects aged 10–80 years. Subsequently, Duane (1922) measured 400 subjects. Turner (1958) measured 1,000 eyes. Turner's values are somewhat lower than Duane and Donders' results because of his method. He moved the target several centimeters closer to the person than the first blur point, then he backed away until the individual reported the first point of clarity. This approach results in lower values.

Research on Accommodation

SYMPTOMS. Many workers have a reduced amplitude of accommodation for their age or accommodative infacility (an inability to quickly change the level of accommodation). These conditions result in blur at near working distances, discomfort, or both (Levine et al., 1985). They also can result in postwork distance blur due to spasm of the accommodative mechanism. The association of accommodative dysfunction with visual symptoms has been shown by Hennessey et al. (1984) and by Levine et al. (1985). The association with other symptoms (general fatigue, concentration difficulties, dizziness, headaches, etc.) has been shown by Jaschinski-Kruza (1991b).

DARK FOCUS OF ACCOMMODATION. The dark focus of accommodation has been researched considerably and is covered extensively in psychological and ergonomic literature. This aspect of accommodation is not as well known among eye care practitioners. Clinical instrumentation for dark focus of accommodation is also not currently available. It is important for eye care practitioners to understand dark focus of accommodation to converse with the ergonomic community.

It has been established that in the absence of visual stimuli (darkness), accommodation and vergence assume "dark" positions that are somewhat closer than infinity. Although there is considerable variation in the dark distances, Owens and Wolf-Kelly (1987) report that the mean dark focus is 67 cm (1.5 D) and the mean dark vergence is 120 cm (0.8-m angles). There is a great deal of individual variation in the dark focus level that is attained, generally ranging from 0.00 to 3.50 D (Jaschinski-Kruza, 1991a). It has been proposed, and with some supporting evidence, that the greatest visual comfort is attained when working at the dark focus or dark vergence position of the eyes; this argument is developed in Chapter 11.

Immediate accommodative history affects the level of dark focus. Ebenholtz (1983) measured the dark focus of accommodation on 12 emmetropes before and after 8-minute fixation periods at the subject's far point and at the subject's near point. The dark focus increased by 0.34 D after near-point fixation and decreased by 0.21 D after far-point fixation. The effects were long lasting—especially after near-point fixation. The effects lasted for hours. Tan and O'Leary (1986) measured the effects of short (5 minutes) and long (1 hour) accommodative stimuli on the dark focus. The stimuli were 0.00 D and 3.00 D. The resting position of accommodation changed in the direction of the stimulus by approximately 0.40 D after the 5-minute stimulus, and it returned to the prestimulus level with a half-life of approximately 15 minutes. After 1 hour of stimulation, the dark focus change remained after 6 hours for two of the subjects. The other two subjects showed a very slow return (half-life of 3 hours) to the original dark focus level.

Jaschinski-Kruza (1991b) measured dark accommodation and psychosomatic complaints on 100 subjects screened for 20/20 vision and to exclude hyperopia. There was a significant correlation between the two—that is, the dark focus was farther away for the group with more symptoms. The symptoms were

1. Tiring more quickly than normal, frequent feelings of fatigue
2. Feelings of listlessness, problems concentrating
3. Dizziness, palpitations of the heart
4. Decreased appetite, vague stomach complaints
5. Sleep disturbances
6. Frequent nervousness, agitation, and headaches

Although the dark focus of accommodation is interesting and offers promise as a clinical test, it has not yet been determined whether measurement of the dark focus of accommodation provides clinically useful information beyond current diagnostic techniques.

ACCOMMODATIVE HYSTERESIS. *Accommodative hysteresis* refers to a change in the tonic level of accommodation, usually as a result of extended viewing at a given distance. The effect is to create a temporary myopia after extended near work. Fisher et al. (1989) showed that the level of accommodative hysteresis was the same whether subjects viewed monocularly or binocularly. This indicates that the convergence system or any accommodative response triggered by the convergence system is not a factor in the amount of accommodative hysteresis.

Gratton et al. (1990) and Gobba et al. (1988) showed that near work causes a change in the resting state of accommodation for distance viewing. After 6 hours of work, 13 out of 14 eyes that were measured showed an increase in myopia (mean increase of 0.19 D) (Gratton et al., 1990). Also, the lag of accommodation as measured at 33 cm increased in 13 of 14 eyes; the average increase in the lag was 0.18 D. Ciuffreda and Ordonez (1995) verified with an autorefractive technique that patients who report a distance blur after near work are, indeed, temporarily myopic.

These studies verify that near work has an effect on tonic accommodation. They support the idea that there is a temporary myopia after near work, which correlates with symptoms of distance blur after extended near work. The studies also support the fact that changes in tonic accommodation are related to other symptoms of visual discomfort.

ACCOMMODATIVE FATIGUE WITH NEAR WORK. Near work, and perhaps computer work in particular, causes at least short-term decreases in accommodative function in some people. Gunnarsson and Soderberg (1983) studied visual changes as a result of work at a cathode ray tube (CRT) in an office setting. They found that the accommodative amplitude decreased after work at a CRT, and that more extensive work resulted in larger decreases. Subjects younger than 35 years had their near point of accommodation recede by an average of 3.5 cm at the end of an intensive day, as opposed to 1.2 cm after a normal day. Ishikawa (1990) studied the accommodative and convergence system in three groups of workers (aged 20–39 years) from the same department: 19 video display terminal (VDT) workers with eyestrain, 12 hard-copy workers with eyestrain (non-VDT), and 19 control subjects without eyestrain who were doing different jobs from the other two groups. All subjects were screened to have low refractive error with 20/20 corrected visual acuity and to have no fixation disparity at distance or near. Objective measurements of accommodative response, pupil response, and convergence were made on Monday morning and on Friday afternoon for all subjects. More abnormal responses were measured in the VDT group (34.6%) than in the non-VDT group (18.5%) and the control group (0%).

Gur and Ron (1992) gave standard eye examinations to 32 VDT workers and 15 non-VDT workers from the same industrial site. They noted a much higher rate of visual impairments in the VDT group—especially deficiencies in fusion and near point of convergence (NPC), heterophoria, amblyopia, and under-corrected ametropia. Then they selected the 16 VDT workers and 13 non-VDT workers who had "no visual defects" (emmetropia with visual acuity of 20/25 or better in each eye, orthophoria, near convergence of 20 prism diopters [PD] or more at near fixation, and near convergence of 10 cm or better). They measured the amplitude of accommodation for all 29 workers at the beginning of the first workday of a week and at the end of the fourth day of a workweek. There was a statistically significant greater loss of accommodation between the two measurements for the VDT group compared to the non-VDT group. The mean decrease for the VDT group was 0.69 D and for the non-VDT group, 0.18 D.

Although it might be intuitively thought that accommodative fatigue responses are due to muscular fatigue, this may not be the case. First of all, the ciliary muscle is smooth muscle, which is generally considered not to fatigue. An alternative explanation has been provided by the work of Lunn and Banks (1986). They found that, after reading text on a VDT, there was a significantly decreased sensitivity to medium spatial frequencies—that is, the detection thresholds were significantly increased. This is apparently the result of the spatial frequency content of the repeating text patterns on the screen. These medium spatial frequencies are critical for proper accommodative response (Charman and Tucker, 1977; Owens, 1980). If, as a result of their tasks, workers become desensitized to the spatial frequencies that drive accommodation, it helps to explain decreased accommodative responses.

IS ACCOMMODATIVE RESPONSE RELATED TO IMAGE QUALITY? Accommodative response becomes more accurate when viewing higher spatial frequencies than when viewing lower ones (Charman and Tucker, 1977). However, Owens (1980) found that the peak for the accommodative response was three to five cycles per degree (intermediate spatial frequencies) and that the accommodative response for gratings of intermediate sinusoidal frequencies was equivalent to the response for a four-cycle-per-degree square-wave grating, which contains the high spatial frequencies. Owens explains that the differences between his findings and those of Charman and Tucker may be due to different instructions given to the subjects. Charman and Tucker's subjects were requested to keep the targets clear, whereas Owens' subjects were simply instructed to view the targets. Charman and Heron (1979) propose that the lower spatial frequencies are used to initiate accommodative responses to a new level, but that the higher spatial frequencies are used to refine the response. They present some measurements to support this theory.

Swan and Richmeier (1997) objectively measured the accommodative response on a group of 17 subjects to printed text and the same text on a computer display (0.26-mm dot pitch), both at a viewing distance of 55 cm. The mean accommodative responses were nearly identical at 1.29 D for the computer display and 1.25 D for paper. They concluded that the monitor they used, which was representative of displays in usage, had sufficient high spatial frequency information to control accommodation as well as the printed page.

It has also been suggested that the images formed by specular reflection from the CRT surface may negatively affect the accommodative response to the display, especially if the specular images are at a distance that could conflict with normal display distance and serve as accommodative stimuli. However, Collins et al. (1994) intensively measured accommodative response on six subjects with the CRT display positioned at 50 cm and specular images of grids and bars at 25 cm. They measured no effect of the reflected images on accommodative response to the display.

Studies have clearly shown that near work, including work at a computer, is strenuous on the accommodative mechanism and results in decreases of the amplitude of accommodation and the frequency of accommodative fluctuations at the end of the day. Most research, however, does not support that viewing a computer screen creates any more of a problem for accommodation than viewing hard copy. This may have been true for earlier computer displays because of poorer resolution, contrast polarity, and contrast; however, current displays are much better than the earlier ones, and it is likely that accommodative response to computer displays is similar to hard copy. However, even with optimum display design, accommodative problems remain a source of symptoms for many patients, whether working at hard copy or computer displays.

Clinical Examination of Accommodation

Certainly an eye examination of a computer worker with symptoms of blur or asthenopia must include an assessment of accommodative functioning. Accommodative assessment must be performed before instillation of mydriatic or cycloplegic pharmaceuticals.

Normal prepresbyopic patients have adequate accommodative abilities to function comfortably at near working distances. However, many workers have a reduced amplitude of accommodation for their age or accommodative infacility (inability to quickly and responsively change the level of accommodation). Sheedy and Parsons (1990) diagnosed 33% of prepresbyopic patients in the Computer Eye Clinic with accommodative disorders, nearly identical to the 34.6% accommodative disorder frequency rate reported in a survey of optometrists (Sheedy, 1992). These accommodative dysfunctions result in blur at near working distances, discomfort, or both. Accommodative dysfunctions also can result in postwork distance blur due to spasm of the accommodative mechanism.

Younger or prepresbyopic individuals can have an improperly functioning accommodative mechanism that results in the symptoms reviewed earlier. The primary tests of accommodative function are shown in Box 5-2. Each test measures a different aspect of accommo-

---

Box 5-2

Clinical tests of accommodation
- Amplitude of accommodation
- Accommodative facility
- Binocular accommodative range (negative relative accommodation/positive relative accommodation)
- Lag of accommodation

dative function, but it is usually not necessary to make all measurements on a given patient.

Amplitude of Accommodation

Method

Usually performed with each eye separately. Slowly move a target with small detail toward the eye. The patient is instructed to note when first detectable blur occurs. Measure the distance from the point of first blur to the spectacle plane in meters; convert to diopters.

The amplitude of accommodation is the most common measurement of accommodation. For normal individuals, the decrease in accommodative amplitude with age is quite predictable. The expected amplitude for different ages can be expressed as $18.5 - 0.3$ (age in years). Expected values are shown in Box 5-3.

Reduced amplitude of accommodation relative to age, in the presence of symptoms, should be considered a possible source of those symptoms.

Box 5-3

Expected amplitude of accommodation with age

Age (yrs)	Amplitude (diopters)
20	12
25	10
30	8–9
35	6–7
40	5–6
45	4

Accommodative Facility

Accommodative facility refers to the ability to quickly change the accommodative response from one level to another. This change in accommodation occurs frequently for computer users who must take information from sheets located at one distance and transfer the information to the computer, with the monitor at another distance.

Hennessey et al. (1984) and Levine et al. (1985) have shown that measures of accommodative facility are related to visual symptoms. Common symptoms are eyestrain; eye fatigue; blur, especially when looking across the room; transcribing errors; and headache.

Accommodative facility is a measure of the ease and quickness with which the accommodation of the eye can change from one accommodative state to another. This test is a very good indicator of accommodative function and should be run on prepresbyopic patients with symptoms.

Method

Patient views target with small detail (20/25) at 40 cm. Quickly interpose ± 1.50 D (or 2.00 D) lenses before the eyes (best performed with hand-held lens flippers [Figure 5-1]), changing the lenses when the patient first notes blur. Measure the number of plus-minus cycles accomplished in 1 minute. The test is usually performed with both eyes open, but it can be performed with each eye independently.

The expected performance for ±1.50 D lenses is 10 cycles per minute with both eyes, and 13 cycles per minute monocularly. For ±2.00 D lenses, the expected values are 11 and 8 cycles per minute. Either 1.50 or 2.00 D lenses can be used with application of the corresponding expected values. Performance with less than the expected values supports diagnosis of accommodative infacility. Performance on this test is often substantially and noticeably reduced. It is often obvious after only two to three cycles that the accommodative response is reduced significantly.

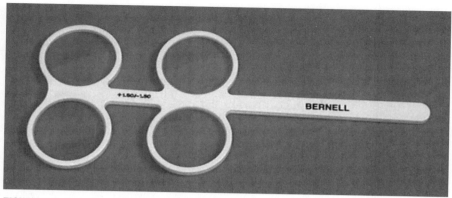

FIGURE 5-1. Lens flippers for accommodative facility testing.

Binocular Accommodative Range
(Negative Relative Range and Positive Relative Range)

Another important indicator of accommodative function is the amount by which accommodation can be binocularly relaxed (with plus lenses) and stimulated (with minus lenses) at a near testing distance (40 cm) and still be able to maintain single clear binocular vision. The plus lens limit is negative relative accommodation (NRA), and the minus lens limit is positive relative accommodation (PRA).

Method

Performed in the phoropter with a 20/25 target at 40 cm with the distance prescription in place. First, plus lenses are inserted in 0.25 D steps until first blur (NRA), and then minus lenses are inserted in 0.25 D steps until first blur (PRA).

This measures the range of accommodative changes that the patient can make and still maintain a single clear image. As such, it is a test of the interaction between accommodation and vergence. For comfortable performance, the NRA-PRA range should be fairly large and well centered (relatively equal values for the NRA and PRA). The NRA and the PRA values should be at least 1.50 D.

Patients with a reduced PRA often have an accommodative disorder or an esophoria; they are averse to accommodating and prefer to relax accommodation. Patients with a reduced NRA are averse to relaxing accommodation and prefer to accommodate more. Frequently, this is an indication of a convergence insufficiency in which the patient wants to accommodate to obtain the accommodative convergence.

Lag of Accommodation

When viewing at near distances, the accommodative response is usually slightly less than the accommodative demand. Because of the depth of focus of the human eye, a near target will be clear although the actual accommodative response is at a slightly farther distance from the eye. The diopter difference between the accommodative demand and the accommodative response is typically 0.50–0.75 D and has been referred to as the "lazy lag of accommodation." Several methods can be used to measure the accommodative lag; dynamic retinoscopy is presented below.

Dynamic retinoscopy method

Can be performed through a phoropter or in free space. The patient binocularly views a detailed near target through the distance prescription with moderate lighting. Perform retinoscopy on one eye while the patient reads the near target. The retinoscope should be located at the same distance from the eye as the reading card and as close to the line of sight as possible. The technique is enhanced by using a near card with a hole in the center for retinoscopy.

The following measurement methods can be applied to the dynamic retinoscopy technique described earlier.

1. Quickly interpose lenses before the eye to determine the lens power required for neutralization of the reflex. The lenses should be interposed quickly to observe the reflex before the accommodative

system can respond to the lens. The lens power required for neutralization is the lag of accommodation.

2. While the patient reads the card, move the retinoscope fore and aft to locate the point of neutrality. Note the distances of the card and the retinoscope neutrality distance; the difference in diopters is the lag of accommodation.

3. Slowly add plus power to both eyes until neutrality is obtained in the plane of the reading card.

The first two methods measure the lag of accommodation. The expected finding is approximately +0.50. Values of +1.00 or greater indicate an excessive lag and accommodative difficulty, perhaps combined with an esophoria (accommodation lags to reduce esophoria). Values of plano or negative indicate over-accommodation, possibly combined with convergence insufficiency (accommodation used to provide convergence).

In the third method, lenses are added slowly so the accommodative system can respond (relaxation to plus lenses). This method does not measure the habitual accommodative lag but rather the amount of plus power to attain accommodative coincidence with the plane of the target. This technique usually results in higher end values, because accommodation decreases or relaxes in response to the plus lenses.

The PRIO unit (Figure 5-2) has been specifically designed for measuring the lag of accommodation using the third method. The front of the instrument simulates a computer screen, and the instrument has a hole in the middle through which the clinician can perform retinoscopy.

Clinical Treatment

Accommodative disorders in the prepresbyopic patient can often be treated with near prescription spectacles or with vision training.

A very effective treatment is to prescribe low plus-power spectacles. These are usually in the range of +0.75 D to +1.25 D over the distance prescription. These spectacles enable the patient to look at the computer screen or other near work without having to use as much accommodation. In effect, low plus lenses lighten the accommodative load on the eye and enable a person to work at near distances more

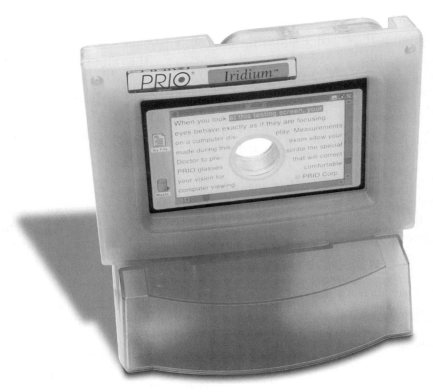

FIGURE 5-2. PRIO device for dynamic retinoscopy.

comfortably. The amount of the near add depends on the severity of the problem. Final power can often best be determined by demonstration to the patient and noting patient response. These single vision glasses blur distant objects, but the amount of the blur is usually tolerable in an office environment. The distance blur should be demonstrated to the patient. If the distance blur is objectionable, then an occupational progressive should be considered (probably selecting a design in which the power digression matches the add you are prescribing), thereby resulting in no add at the top of the lens (see Occupational Progressive Addition Lenses in Chapter 6).

Vision training can often improve the amplitude of accommodation and facility of accommodation up to age-expected performance. Bobier and Sivak (1983), Liu et al. (1979), and Daum (1983) have all demonstrated the efficacy of visual training at resolving accommodative problems. The techniques used vary from practitioner to practitioner, but, most commonly, the training program largely involves one office session per week accompanied by daily home exercises that should be performed on a regular basis (i.e., three 10-minute sessions each day). Usually, 10–15 sessions are adequate.

Whether a particular patient's problem is treated by vision training or spectacles (or both) depends on the nature of the accommodative problem, the patient's time availability, and the preferences of the doctor and patient in treatment methodology. However, spectacle treatment is often the quicker and less expensive option, especially considering that many computer workers do not have the time to commit to a training program.

Binocular Vision

Although most people keep their eyes aligned when viewing an object, many individuals have a heterophoria and difficulty maintaining alignment. This causes symptoms such as fatigue, headache, blur, double vision, and general ocular discomfort. Heterophoria is measured by interrupting binocular fusion and measuring eye alignment in the absence of fusion. The diagrams in Figure 5-3 depict the conditions of orthophoria, esophoria, and exophoria. These are the conditions in which the occluded eye respectively remains aligned, moves inward, or moves outward relative to the normal alignment position.

In the presence of heterophoria, constant neuromuscular effort is required to keep the eyes aligned. Whether a person experiences symptoms depends on the amount of the misalignment, the ability of the individual to overcome that misalignment, and the difficulty of the task. The symptoms associated with heterophoria are eyestrain, double vision, headaches, eye irritation, and general fatigue. Clinical studies have documented the relationships between the visual clinical measurements of binocular vision and symptoms (Sheedy and Saladin, 1977, 1978, 1983).

Eye alignment at near viewing distances is more complex than at distance because of the ocular convergence required to view near

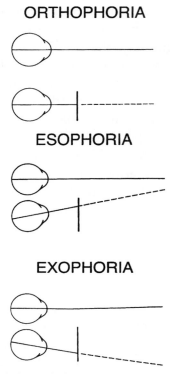

FIGURE 5-3. Orthophoria, esophoria, exophoria.

objects and because of the interaction between the ocular convergence and accommodative mechanisms. Treatment of these conditions can include refractive or prismatic correction or vision training exercises.

Convergence

To maintain binocular fixation on objects that are at closer viewing distances, it is necessary to converge, or "cross," the eyes. One of the most common clinical methods to quantify convergence ability is to determine the closest distance to which one can converge one's eyes. This is called the NPC and is recorded in centimeters. Patients with a poor convergence ability have a convergence insufficiency. This commonly results in symptoms of eyestrain and eye fatigue (Grisham, 1988).

The literature on the incidence of convergence insufficiency was reviewed by Bennett et al. (1982). The studies show that 10–30% of adults have convergence insufficiency. However, the criteria for arriving at this diagnosis are not uniform across studies. Grieve and Archibald (1942) measured the NPC on 1,268 healthy adult males (military recruits). They determined 884 subjects (69.7%) with full voluntary convergence of closer than 8 cm, 147 (11.6%) with "imperfect voluntary convergence" of 8–12 cm, and 237 (18.7%) "without voluntary convergence" of greater than 12 cm.

Convergence insufficiency is quite common in the population as a whole. People who do not perform demanding near visual work do not develop symptoms from their convergence insufficiency. Frequently, it seems as if people with convergence insufficiency have occupations, lifestyles, or both in which they seldom view materials at near distances. It is a clinical impression that these people (and those with other near point visual problems) may have designed their life around their visual difficulties, perhaps beginning at a very early age. However, because work at a computer has become integral to many jobs today, it appears that many people with convergence insufficiency are required to use their near vision and, hence, have the ensuing symptoms.

Older adults commonly experience convergence insufficiency because of the increase in exophoria at near with the increase in bifocal power. Often they say, "I used to love to read for hours, but now I grow tired and fall asleep after only 10 minutes." The convergence insufficiency problem can be further exacerbated by the need for high adds in patients with reduced acuity due to conditions such as cataract or macular degeneration. The closer viewing distances required by such high adds place a greater demand on convergence.

Dark Vergence

As with the dark focus of accommodation, the dark vergence position is determined by placing the subject in the dark (no fusional or accommodative stimulus) and determining the vergence position of the eyes. Also, as with dark accommodation, dark vergence is better known in the ergonomic community, and no clinical test is available.

There is evidence that symptoms of discomfort are related more to vergence problems (as measured with the dark vergence position) than to accommodative problems. Owens and Wolf-Kelly (1987) found that subjective ratings of visual discomfort were significantly related to dark vergence changes, but not to the dark focus changes. This is also supported by the work of Jaschinski-Kruza (1988). He had two groups of individuals (one with a dark focus of 50 cm, and one with a dark focus of 100 cm) perform VDT work. Both groups preferred the 100-cm viewing distance and reported less strain at this distance. Both groups had a far dark vergence; therefore, the preferred viewing distance correlated with the dark vergence position and not with the dark accommodation. However, the visual strain at the 50-cm position was lower in the near dark focus group than in the far dark focus group. Jaschinski-Kruza (1991a) also found that visual strain at a 50-cm VDT task was related to the dark vergence position—the farther the dark vergence position, the greater the eyestrain.

Tyrrell and Leibowitz (1990) measured the dark vergence position on 104 persons and found that it was significantly related to visual symptoms—that is, it was farther away in those individuals with symptoms. In a second experiment, they screened 16 subjects to have a clear "Heuer effect." This is the effect whereby the dark vergence position is farther away with a higher gaze position (20 degrees upward) compared to a lower gaze position (20 degrees downward). They read at a distance of 20 cm at both 20 degrees above and below the neutral position of 5.1 degrees downward. More visual symptoms were reported in the up gaze position, thereby supporting the idea that symptoms are related to the difference between the vergence position of the task and the dark vergence position. However, other possible differences between upper and lower gaze positions cannot be ruled out.

As with the dark focus of accommodation, the dark vergence position is not measured (per se) in the clinic. Dark focus and dark vergence are measurements that have been used in research experiments, but their relationships to common clinical measurements have not been studied. In fact, there appears to be a lack of communication between the researchers and the clinicians in this regard. It is not known whether these dark measurements provide useful information that adds to the use of current clinical data.

In particular, the dark vergence position of the eyes is extremely similar to the phoria measurement that is commonly determined in clinical examinations—the only difference is whether the patient is viewing into the dark or whether he or she is viewing a fixation target with fusion denied. It would be useful to know how the phoria measurement relates to the dark vergence position. If there is any difference between them, the distance phoria might seem to be related more to the operating conditions of the visual system than to the dark focus. Also, the near phoria measurement of the eyes includes the effects of accommodative convergence and has been shown to be a clinically useful tool with strong relationships to symptoms (see Clinical Diagnosis). The dark vergence position of the eyes would appear to offer less information than the distance and the near phorias, measurements that are of proven use and are in common clinical use.

If dark focus of accommodation and dark vergence are to be used clinically, their usefulness with respect to current clinical techniques must first be shown, and then methods and instruments must be developed to enable their measurement in a clinical setting.

Clinical Diagnosis

In a retrospective study of patients examined in the Computer Eye Clinic, Sheedy and Parsons (1990) reported clinically significant esophoria and exophoria in approximately one-third of the prepresbyopic population of patients. As with accommodative disorders, this is a greater percentage than has been reported in other adult age populations. Again, this is probably a reflection of the high near-point demands of computer tasks.

The binocular vision, or alignment status, can be different at different viewing distances. Certainly, it can be very different at infinity (greater than 4 m) from what it is at close viewing distances (40 cm). By convention and tradition, 40 cm is the standard distance at which the near vision is assessed. As a result, nearly all of the clinical data, experience, and research are for measurements at this working dis-

---

Box 5-4

Effective clinical measures of binocular vision

- Phoria
- Vergence ranges
- Near point of convergence
- Fixation disparity
- Vergence facility

---

tance. A good argument can be made that for computer users who are viewing at 50–60 cm, the visual testing should be made at those distances. Although this argument is persuasive, it is probably more sensible to perform the near testing at 40 cm, in which experience and the research database provide support. Although the accommodative and convergence demands are somewhat less at 50–60 cm than at 40 cm, the same factors are at play at all of these distances. A diagnosed binocular vision problem at 40 cm almost certainly indicates a binocular vision problem at the 50- to 70-cm viewing distances for the computer screen—and most computer workers also perform considerable near work at the typical 40-cm distance. Therefore, the position taken here is to examine at 40 cm, and then refine with measurements at a different distance if indicated (Box 5-4).

It is important for the clinician to understand the relationships between asthenopic symptoms and the various measures of oculomotor coordination so that he or she can accurately analyze the clinical data to diagnose the condition and determine whether oculomotor coordination problems are causative of the symptoms. Sheedy and Saladin (1977, 1978) measured phoria, vergence, and fixation disparity curves on populations of symptomatic and asymptomatic individuals and determined the clinical measures that were the best discriminators between the two populations. The results are used in the following suggestions for clinical measurement and interpretation.

PHORIA

Method

The preferred method is prism neutralization of the cover test with the patient viewing a target with small detail at 40 cm. An alternative method is the von Graefe technique through the phoropter—vertical disassociating prism before one eye and using horizontal measuring prism before the other eye to obtain vertical alignment of the double images.

The phoria is a measure of the latent alignment of the eyes when sensory fusion is denied. The phoria measurement is usually made at distance (greater than 4 m) and also at near (most commonly at 40 cm). The near measurement is most relevant to computer-using patients. Small amounts of exophoria are normal (Sheedy and Saladin, 1983) (i.e., 0–6 PD). Exophoria larger than this can be associated with convergence insufficiency. Measurements of prism-induced vergences and the NPC are indicated with larger exophorias. Esophoria is much less compatible with comfortable vision than is exophoria. Any amount of esophoria in a patient with visually related symptoms should be considered suspect.

VERGENCES

Method

Perform in phoropter using a small, detailed target at 40 cm. Use a rotary prism to slowly add base-in prism equally in the two eyes. Note and record the amount of prism when the patient reports first noticeable blur and first fusional break. Then, reduce the prism and note prism value at first recovery of fusion. Repeat with base-out prism.

The vergences are a measure of the range of vergence angles through which sensory fusion can maintain alignment of the eyes. In general, the vergence range should be quite large and well centered for comfortable vision.

SHEARD'S CRITERION. Sheard's criterion is often used to determine whether the phoria and vergences are adequate. Sheard's criterion is that the opposing vergence should be twice the size of the phoria magnitude for comfort. In studies of symptomatic populations compared to asymptomatic populations of patients and subjects (Sheedy and Saladin, 1977, 1978), Sheard's criterion was the single best discriminator between the symptomatic and asymptomatic groups—but only for those with exophoria. Sheard's criterion did not discriminate for patients with esophoria. Therefore, when analyzing an exophoria, it is valuable to determine if the positive vergence (to the blur point) is twice the value of the exophoria. It is not useful to make this determination in the case of esophoria.

Inherent to Sheard's criterion is the concept that the opposing vergence overcomes or stabilizes the phoria deviation. Sheard's usefulness for exophoria supports the contention that positive vergences are used to overcome an exophoria; by contrast, the concept of negative vergences overcoming an esophoria is erroneous. This is consistent with the fact that positive vergences are an active process, whereas negative vergences are more passive.

NEAR POINT OF CONVERGENCE

Method

Slowly bring a small near object toward the bridge of the nose. Encourage the patient to maintain fusion as close as possible. Note the distance in centimeters from the point of convergence release to the center of ocular rotation. Repeat three times. Also note any subjective strain or discomfort in performing the test.

The NPC is a critical measure to determine if there is a convergence insufficiency and should be measured on all patients with near point symptoms. An NPC of greater than 8 cm is suspect. However, even if the patient is able to converge to 2–3 cm, convergence insufficiency is not necessarily ruled out. Repeated measure of the NPC sometimes results in a dramatic increase in the measure. The patient's subjective response during the test should also be carefully observed. Many patients demonstrate obvious discomfort while crossing their eyes. For these patients, hold the target close to their NPC for 10 seconds. Afterwards, ask if they felt uncomfortable (they obviously did!). Then ask whether the strain they feel is similar to the symptoms they experience at work. A positive response (which often follows) confirms the diagnosis in the view of the doctor and the patient. Because the treatment of choice for convergence insufficiency is visual training, this also serves to convince and motivate the patient to perform the training.

VERTICAL PHORIA. The vertical phoria should be routinely measured with Maddox rod, von Graefe technique, cover test, or other methods. If a vertical phoria is determined, it should be verified with a second technique. The vertical vergence range or vertical fixation disparity can also be helpful in this determination. A vertical phoria of 1.0 PD (certainly) and even 0.5 PD can cause generalized asthenopic symptoms. Other symptoms can be disorientation or losing one's place while reading.

STRABISMUS AND OTHER OCULOMOTOR DYSFUNCTIONS. Frequently, individuals with strabismus are effective at suppressing the vision in the eye not looking at the object and have no particular symptoms associated with their condition when working at the computer. However, some individuals with a strabismus have difficulties associated with their condition, and these should be fully investigated and treated when possible. A strabismic individual who usually suppresses the vision in one eye can have difficulty suppressing at the computer. This can occur especially with a dark background computer screen that is surrounded by a bright environment, which makes it more difficult to suppress the vision of the unaligned eye. It can be helpful to ensure that the luminance ratios are not excessive in the work environment for this patient (see Chapter 8).

Sometimes it is difficult to determine whether the strabismus (or another binocular vision problem) is causing the patient's symptoms. In these cases, consider giving the patient a patch that the patient should wear long enough and often enough to determine whether monocular occlusion eliminates the symptoms. A positive response confirms that binocular vision is a source of the symptoms.

Difficulty with saccadic or smooth pursuit movement disorders can also be problematic for computer users. These disorders can contribute to fixation problems, poor performance, and symptoms. Such conditions are often secondary to accommodative and binocular vision disorders.

FINAL DIAGNOSIS OF LATERAL ALIGNMENT. Heterophoria is extremely common, and the existence of heterophoria, by itself, does not indicate a problem with binocular vision. The clinical challenge is to determine whether the particular heterophoria in a given patient is causing or contributing to the patient's symptoms.

Exophoria problems are characterized by relatively high exophoria, poor positive vergences, and, often, a reduced NPC. It is also common to have a reduced NRA and a strong PRA; this is because the patient may require more accommodation to obtain convergence through accommodation.

Eso problems are characterized by an esophoria (even small amounts), a relatively large accommodative lag, and a low PRA. The accommodative lag and the poor PRA are results of the patient being more comfortable and able to relax accommodation because accommodative convergence makes the patient more eso. Although accommodative disorders can be independent of binocular alignment problems, it is common for patients with eso problems to also have accommodative problems (Box 5-5).

Clinical Treatment

The most common successful treatments for binocular vision problems are easier to outline than are their diagnoses (Box 5-6).

Exo conditions and convergence insufficiency, which often accompany one another, are usually best treated with vision training. Exophoric patients must continuously cross their eyes to keep them aligned. The condition is treated by training the patients to cross their eyes more efficiently and comfortably. Patient motivation and handling are essential for successful treatment. It is fortuitous that the convergence mechanism (eye-crossing) is the most easily trainable function in

Box 5-5

Diagnostic criteria for clinically significant heterophoria

Exophoria	**Esophoria**	**Vertical phoria**
• Small amounts of exophoria are expected, more than 10 prism diopters at greater risk for problems • Positive vergences do not meet Sheard's criterion • Reduced near point of convergence • Reduced negative relative accommodation	• Even small amounts of esophoria can be problematic • Large accommodative lag • Reduced positive relative accommodation	• 0.5 Prism diopter can be significant • Asymmetric vertical vergences • Vertical fixation disparity

Box 5-6

Common treatment of binocular vision disorders

Diagnosis	**Treatment**
Exophoria problem, convergence insufficiency	Convergence training
Esophoria problem	Reading add
Vertical phoria	Prism

the visual system. Most cases of convergence insufficiency can be successfully treated in 5–15 weeks, depending on complications and patient motivation and compliance. Refractive power lenses or prism are not usually successful in treating exo conditions. A typical therapy program consists of a weekly office visit with daily home-oriented therapy. Suggested home training exercises are shown in Figure 5-4.

Plus lenses exacerbate the exophoria, and minus lenses may help the exophoria but create a greater demand on accommodation—a demand that adult computer workers cannot afford. Base-in prism, which could assist the exophoria at near, usually creates an esophoria at distance. Although the glasses may be designed for only near distances, the patient will view distant objects through them, and the effect of an unaccustomed esophoria when glancing at distance is unacceptable.

Eso conditions are most successfully treated with plus lenses for near that reduce or eliminate the esophoria by relaxing accommodative convergence. The plus prescription can be in a single vision pair of glasses or a multifocal (see Chapter 6). Vision training can be a successful alternative treatment for eso conditions.

Vertical phoria problems should be treated with a prism prescription; there is no other successful alternative.

Chapter 6 explores how to successfully diagnose and treat patients whose accommodation has been compromised by presbyopia.

Action Items

1. Determine which accommodation or binocular tests, or both, you will add to your computer-user examination.
2. What criteria will you use to diagnose accommodative and binocular disorders?
3. Determine how you will use accommodative and binocular vision test results for prescribing near lenses for prepresbyopic patients.
4. Develop office policies and procedures on handling patients with accommodative and binocularity disorders, including scripts for what to say to the patient, demonstrations of the disorder, and visual therapy to correct.
5. Train staff to provide the appropriate visual therapy prescribed.

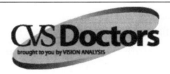

Vision Training—Convergence

1. Push-up: High sustained

   Equipment: Near point target—can use finger.

   Slowly bring the object as close to the eyes as possible while maintaining fusion. Hold it for at least 10 seconds. Patient should feel the strain in his or her eyes.

   Goals: Bring the target as close as possible. Hold the target for longer periods.

2. Push-up: Far-near rock

   Equipment: Near point target—can use finger.

   Slowly bring the object as close to the eyes as possible while maintaining fusion. Keep the object at this position and look past it at a distant (at least 10 ft) object. Look back and forth between the distant and the near object at least 10 times. Patient should feel the strain in his or her eyes. Patient should also be aware of two objects going into one when switching distances.

   Goals: Bring the target as close as possible. Perform more cycles. Perform the exercise faster.

3. Push-up: Combination

   This is a combination of Nos. 1 and 2 above. Patient first performs No. 1 for 10 seconds and then immediately goes into No. 2 without stopping or changing the position of the near target.

4. Prism jump

   Equipment: Hand-held prism—amount (4–12 prism diopters [PD]) selected by doctor. Near fixation target.

   Patient views the near target at usual reading distance. The patient interposes the prism (base-out or with the fat part toward the outside of the face) before one eye. Patient should note two objects going into one. Remove prism and, again, note two objects going into one. Perform at least 10 cycles of prism in and out.

   Goals: Increase speed, prism amount, and number of cycles.

5. Far-near rock with prism

FIGURE 5-4. Convergence insufficiency—home training exercises.

Equipment: Hand-held prism—amount (4–12 PD) selected by doctor. Near fixation target.

Patient places prism before one eye (base-out or with the fat part toward the outside of the face) and views back and forth between a distant object and the near object placed at usual reading distance. Patient should be aware of two objects going into one when switching distances. Perform at least 10 cycles.

Variation: Remove prism when looking at distance, interpose prism when looking at near.

Goals: Increase speed, prism amount, and number of cycles.

6. Prism reading

Equipment: Hand-held prism—amount (4–12 PD) selected by doctor. Reading material.

Patient places prism before one eye and reads usual reading material.

Variation 1: Continuous reading with base-out or with the fat part toward the outside of the face.

Variation 2: Alternate pages (or paragraphs) with and without the prism.

Variation 3: Alternate pages (or paragraphs) with base-out and base-in prism.

Goals: Increase prism amount and increase reading time.

7. Lens flippers

Equipment: Lens flippers—amount (±1.00 to ±2.50) selected by doctor. Near fixation target with detail.

View detailed target at usual reading distance. Interpose one set of lenses. As soon as the target becomes refocused, switch the lenses. Repeat. Perform at least 10 cycles.

Goals: Increase speed, number of cycles, and lens strength.

8. Flipper reading

Equipment: Lens flippers—amount (±1.00 to ±2.50) selected by doctor. Usual reading material.

Variation 1: Read the usual reading material through the minus lenses.

Variation 2: Alternate pages (or paragraphs) with and without the minus lenses.

Variation 3: Alternate pages (or paragraphs) with plus and minus lenses.

FIGURE 5-4. (Continued)

References

Bennett GR, Blondin M, Ruskiewicz J. Incidence and prevalence of selected visual conditions. J Am Optom Assoc 1982;53(8):647–656.

Bobier WR, Sivak JG. Orthoptic treatment of subjects showing slow accommodative responses. Am J Optom Physiol Opt 1983;60(8):678–687.

Borish I. Clinical Refraction (3rd ed). Chicago: Professional Press, 1970.

Charman WN, Heron G. Spatial frequency and the dynamics of the accommodation response. Optica Acta 1979;26(2):217–228.

Charman WN, Tucker J. Dependence of accommodation response on the spatial frequency spectrum of the observed object. Vision Res 1977;17:129–139.

Ciuffreda KJ, Ordonez X. Abnormal transient myopia in symptomatic individuals after sustained near work. Optom Vis Sci 1995;72(7):506–510.

Collins M, Davis B, Atchison D. VDT screen reflections and accommodative response. Ophthalmic Physiol Opt 1994;14(2):193–198.

Daum KM. Accommodative insufficiency. Am J Optom Physiol Opt 1983;60:352–359.

Donders FC. On the anomalies of accommodation and refraction of the eye. London: The New Sydenham Society, 1864.

Duane A. Studies in monocular and binocular accommodation with their clinical applications. Am J Ophthalmol 1922;5:865.

Ebenholtz SM. Accommodative hysteresis: a precursor for induced myopia? Invest Ophthalmol Vis Sci 1983;24:513–515.

Fisher SK, Ciuffreda KJ, Bird JE. The effect of monocular versus binocular fixation on accommodative hysteresis. Ophthalmic Physiol Opt 1989;8:438–442.

Gobba FM, Broglia A, Sarti R, et al. Visual fatigue in video display terminal operators: objective measure and relation to environmental conditions. Int Arch Occup Environ Health 1988;60:81–87.

Gratton I, Piccoli B, Zaniboni A, et al. Change in visual function and viewing distance during work with VDTs. Ergonomics 1990;33(12):1433–1441.

Grieve J, Archibald DH. Some facts and figures relating to heterophoria in symptom-free individuals. Trans Ophthalmol Soc U K 1942;62:285–295.

Grisham JD. Visual therapy results for convergence insufficiency: a literature review. Am J Optom Physiol Opt 1988;65(6):448–454.

Gunnarsson E, Soderberg I. Eye strain resulting from VDU work at the Swedish Telecommunications Administration. Appl Ergon 1983;14:61–69.

Gur S, Ron S. Does work with visual display units impair visual activities after work? Doc Ophthalmol 1992:79:253–259.

Hennessey D, Iosue RA, Rouse MW. Relation of symptoms to accommodative infacility of school aged children. Am J Optom Physiol Opt 1984;61(3):177–183.

Ishikawa S. Examination of the near triad in VDU operators. Ergonomics 1990; 33(6):787–798.

Jaschinski-Kruza W. Visual strain during VDU work: the effect of viewing distance and dark focus. Ergonomics 1988;31(10):1449–1465.

Jaschinski-Kruza W. Eyestrain in VDU users: viewing distance and the resting position of ocular muscles. Hum Factors 1991a;33(1):69–83.

Jaschinski-Kruza W. Relations between dark accommodation and psychosomatic symptoms. Ophthalmic Physiol Opt 1991b;12:103–105.

Levine S, Ciuffreda KJ, Selenow A, Flax N. Clinical assessment of accommodative ability in symptomatic and asymptomatic individuals. J Am Optom Assoc 1985;56(4):286–290.

Liu JS, Lee M, Jang J, Ciuffreda KJ, et al. Objective assessment of accommodation orthoptics. 1. Dynamic insufficiency. Am J Optom Physiol Opt 1979;56(5):285–294.

Lunn R, Banks WP. Visual fatigue and spatial frequency adaptation to video displays of text. Hum Factors 1986;28(4):457–464.

Owens DA. A comparison of accommodative responsiveness and contrast sensitivity for sinusoidal gratings. Vision Res 1980;20:159–167.

Owens DA, Wolf-Kelly K. Near work, visual fatigue, and variations of oculomotor tonus. Invest Ophthalmol Vis Sci 1987;28(4):743–749.

Sheedy JE. Vision problems at video display terminals: a survey of optometrists. J Am Optom Assoc 1992;63:687–692.

Sheedy JE, Parsons SP. The video display terminal eye clinic: clinical report. Optom Vis Sci 1990;67(8):622–626.

Sheedy JE, Saladin JJ. Phoria, vergence and fixation disparity in oculomotor problems. Am J Optom Physiol Opt 1977;54(7):474–478.

Sheedy JE, Saladin JJ. Association of symptoms with measures of oculomotor deficiencies. Am J Optom Physiol Opt 1978;55(10):670–676.

Sheedy JE, Saladin JJ. Validity of diagnostic criteria and case analysis in binocular vision disorders. In C Schor, K Ciuffreda (eds), Basic and Clinical Aspects of Binocular Vergence Eye Movements. Boston: Butterworth, 1983;517–540.

Swan S, Richmeier K. Accommodation to text and VDT displays. Optom Vis Sci 1997;74(12s):182.

Tan RKT, O'Leary DJ. Stability of the accommodative dark focus after periods of maintained accommodation. Invest Ophthalmol Vis Sci 1986;27:1414–1417.

Turner MJ. Observations of the normal subjective amplitude of accommodation. Br J Physiol Opt 1958;15(2):70–100.

Tyrrell RA, Leibowitz HW. The relation of vergence effort to reports of visual fatigue following prolonged near work. Hum Factors 1990;32(3):341–357.

6
Presbyopia and Computer Use

Presbyopia is the condition that results when the normal age-related loss of accommodation prevents the patient from comfortably maintaining focus on near objects. The usual treatment for presbyopia is to prescribe reading glasses or multifocal lenses. The power of the lenses that are prescribed for a presbyope depends on how much remaining accommodation the person has and the distance that the person needs to see clearly. Once a person reaches the age of 60 years, accommodation has essentially been reduced to zero, and the lens power is almost completely based on the distance the patient needs to see clearly.

The most common method for prescribing and designing multifocals for general wear (e.g., progressive addition lenses [PALs] or bifocals) is to prescribe a lens power that provides clear vision at 40 cm (16 in.); this is the standard testing distance used by eye doctors. PALs and bifocals prescribed for general wear also have the near power located so that 25–30 degrees of ocular depression is required to view through the near addition. The most common corrections for presbyopia are designed to provide clear vision at 40 cm with a downward gaze angle of 25–30 degrees.

The most common problem for presbyopic computer users is that the normal glasses that meet their visual needs for most other tasks usually do not properly correct their vision for the computer display. The computer display is usually farther away (50–70 cm or 20–28 in.) than the usual reading distance for which the multifocal glasses have been prescribed (40 cm). Also, the computer display is higher (10–20 degrees downward) than where the lens addition is (25–30 degrees downward). A presbyope who tries to wear his or her "usual" multifocal correction at the computer either does not see the computer display clearly or needs to assume an awkward posture, resulting in neck and back strain. Most commonly, presbyopes need to inch closer to the screen and tilt their heads backward; the former is bad for the back, and the latter is bad for the neck. This is true for bifocal lenses and PALs. Although PALs provide a region with an intermediate add, this is the portion of the lens with the narrowest field of clear vision. The person wearing PALs must continually find the small sweet spot on the lens and use his or her neck to move the head rather than moving the eyes.

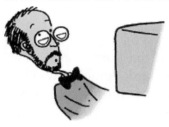

Many, if not most, computer workers who require multifocals for normal visual tasks also require a separate pair of spectacles for their computer work. It is very helpful to the eye doctor for computer workers to measure the distance from their eyes to the computer display and to reference documents and also to note the height of these things relative to their eyes. This information should be brought with them to their eye examination because it influences the prescription.

Prescription Determination and Lens Design

Prescribing for presbyopia is second nature to any eye doctor, but special considerations need be given to prescribing for the presbyopic computer user. It usually requires a different prescription and lens design from those that meet the other daily visual needs of the patient.

For general eyewear prescriptions, the prescription determination and the spectacle design are usually determined in two separate steps; for computer-using patients, it is best to determine the prescription and design together.

Where Is the Computer and Other Work?

To properly prescribe lenses for a person in the presbyopic years, it is useful to know how far the computer display is from the eyes and also how far other near work is from the patient's eyes. In many cases, this information is required to determine the correct prescription or lens design or to enable counseling about workstation arrangement or changes.

The viewing distance and height of the computer screen can be obtained by sending an advance questionnaire (as mentioned in Chapter 2) to the patient. It can also be obtained by sending the patient back to his or her workplace and determining the final prescription and spectacle design on a return visit. Patients are not very good at reconstructing this information without making direct measurements.

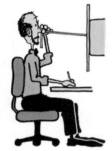

It is not always prudent to prescribe for the viewing distance and angle of the patient's current computer location. This is because the patient's current conditions may be compromised due to poor workstation arrangement or an existing eye condition (e.g., a person having a much longer than typical viewing distance because of uncorrected presbyopia). A reason should be determined if the viewing distance is outside the range of 20–28 in. (50–70 cm) or if the center of the screen is outside the range of 4–9 in. below the eyes.

In some cases, the screen may be legitimately or necessarily located outside of these ranges. For example, the person may be operating with a very large screen with large images or text or without a requirement to see small detail. In such a case, it can be very appropriate (probably advantageous) to work at a much longer viewing distance. Some workstations enable the worker to assume a reclined position. This is common for people who spend many continuous hours at a workstation. If they recline, it is necessary that they have head support (a head rest). Reclining also usually results in the computer screen being higher than the eyes. When prescribing for these people, the backward head tilt needs to be considered in the design of any multifocal. In some cases, a particularly short viewing distance is required if seeing small detail is required (e.g., desktop publishing during layout). In such cases, however, it is important to counsel the patient to bring the computer toward him- or herself rather than leaning forward to see the computer. In some cases, the computer location is fixed by the workstation and the patient has no control over changing it. In all of these "legitimate" reasons for the computer location being outside of normal ranges, it is appropriate to prescribe the lens addition and lens design to meet the current location of the computer.

However, in many other cases, an unusual computer location indicates a problem that should or can be fixed before prescribing. Some patients who are "fighting" the onset of presbyopia have learned to push their computer away from them. Patients with myopia in the range of 2.00–3.50 diopters (D) may be taking their glasses off for computer work and, therefore, working at a distance that is too short. Computer screen locations that are too high are common, especially for shorter people. If the screen is too high and the patient has an upright posture at the computer, then he or she should be counseled about lowering the computer screen. This can often be accomplished by removing the computer from atop the central processing unit. Computer locations that are too low can easily be made higher with spacers—a phone book often works well.

If the current screen location is appropriate or if it cannot be altered, then this information can be used for prescribing. If not, then the prescription should be designed for the altered location of the computer screen.

If specific information about the computer location is not available, it is probably best to design the prescription and lenses for a 60-cm (24-in.) viewing distance and a screen center located 15 cm (6 in.) below eye level. This assumption has a greater likelihood of being valid if the person is working at a fairly standard computer workstation for word processing. However, many workstations have visual requirements that are significantly different from this arrangement, especially for special applications.

Determining the Addition for the Computer Display

In some cases, beginning presbyopes are able to use their normal glasses at the computer, because they do not yet require an add for the intermediate distance and are using the distance portion of their glasses. This can be the case if they have bifocals or PALs. However, once a patient begins to require an add for the computer viewing distance, his or her usual correction is seldom acceptable.

It is very common for a presbyopic individual to require his or her first near correction for computer work, although the computer viewing distance is farther from the eyes than most other near tasks, and it might be expected that this task would not require a correction until later in life. This may be because of the extended near viewing that is often required by work at a computer and also because of the fact that most computer users also need to see at normal reading distances for part of their workday. It is very common for patients who would normally be considered prepresbyopic to require a near prescription at their computer. These patients can be in their thirties and often exhibit a reduced amplitude of accommodation for their age or poor accommodative facility. A near prescription can be very successful at improving their function and comfort at the computer.

Final prescription determination (add power) is often best determined by demonstration. For advanced presbyopia, the required add for the computer distance is usually 0.50–0.75 of that required for 40 cm. A straight calculation based on the 40-cm add often does not work for various reasons. It is important to determine the needed add at the viewing distance of the computer and to measure the range of clear distances through the add. Demonstration to the patient is important.

The measurements and demonstration can be made with a card on the near point rod of the phoropter, although some near point rods are not long enough to enable testing at longer computer-viewing distances. It is often very effective to make the final prescription measurement in free space by seating patients at a computer workstation and using a meter stick to locate their eyes at their usual distance. Simulated computer screens, including the PRIO unit, are available to serve this purpose. This also reminds your patients about the special care they are receiving for their computer work. Lens flippers can be very useful to quickly demonstrate different add levels. In combination or separately, lens flippers can be used over the patient's old prescription or distance prescription in a trial frame to demonstrate different adds and to measure working distance ranges.

The patient's intermediate needs, near viewing needs, and distance viewing needs should be determined by history, and the prescription and lens design determined accordingly. Although the primary visual needs are at the intermediate distance, nearly all computer users also have some viewing requirements at 40 cm. Distance visual needs are often considerably less important and can often be compromised in the interests of best meeting the intermediate and near needs.

Now you have the distance refractive correction, the normal 40 cm add, and the add required for the computer. The prescription that is written depends on the lens design selected for the patient.

Single Vision Lenses

Younger presbyopic computer users are often successfully fitted with single vision lenses designed for the computer distance. This is because they have enough remaining accommodation to see clearly at 40 cm with the add for the computer distance (nearly all computer users still have extensive viewing needs at 40 cm). In demonstrating the add, it is important to measure the range of clear vision to ensure that it also includes the patient's near visual needs if you are considering prescribing single vision lenses. In most of these cases, an add of +0.75 to +1.25 is appropriate. If it is possible to accomplish without compromising the patient's near vision, trim the add on the low side to decrease the distance blur.

The distance blur through this single vision prescription should be demonstrated to the patient. For most patients, the distance blur is acceptable because their distance visual needs in the office are limited, and the amount of blur created by the relatively low add is small. Usually, vision for conversation with others and for walking around the immediate confines of the office is good. However, if the distance blur is disturbing to the patient, another design is indicated.

A single vision correction offers the advantages of a large, clear field of vision, and it is also the least costly alternative.

Occupational Progressive Addition Lenses

Occupational progressive lenses are specially designed lenses that often can meet the presbyopic patient's computer vision needs very successfully, especially for those patients who wear PALs for general wear. In fact, most PAL wearers would find it unacceptable to wear a pair of bifocals. Clinical trials support the acceptance of occupational progressives by computer users (Bachman, 1992; Brischer et al., 1994; Hanks et al., 1996; Butzon and Eagles, 1997). Most major lens manufacturers have a lens design in this category. These lenses are seamless (i.e., they are based on PAL technology) and are designed to provide the appropriate add power for the required viewing angles in the computer environment. All of the lenses provide the full near add (40 cm) in the bottom of the lens. The central portion of the lens provides an intermediate power for the patient, and the add power generally declines further toward the top of the lens. This allows patients to look up and see at farther distances in their office environment. However, the top of the lens typically does not include the distance refractive correction (except the Technica [American Optical, Southbridge, MA] and Tact [Hoya, Bethel, CT], which provide a small area containing the distance correction).

For the convenience of the practitioner, these lenses are prescribed by writing the usual distance prescription with the usual 40-cm add, and then specifying the lens design from those available (see Table 6-1 for the occupational lens designs). The lenses are characterized by having a lens power degression (i.e., the amount by which the add power decreases from the bottom to the top of the lens). The prescribed near power is provided in the bottom of the lens (this is the power to which the optical laboratory finishes the lens), and the power in the top of the lens is determined by the lens degression. In nearly all cases, there is some remaining add in the top of the lens. The available degressions for each lens are listed in Table 6-1.

Some clinicians can be successful by using just one or two of the lens designs. It can be very effective to simply write the usual distance-near prescription and specify the occupational lens of choice. For lens

TABLE 6-1. Occupational progressive lenses

Name	Manufacturer	Degression powers
Access	SOLA, Petaluma, CA	0.75, 1.25
Cosmolit Office	Rodenstock, Columbus, OH	0.75, 1.25
Gradal RD	Zeiss, Chester, VA	0, top is +0.50 add
Interview	Essilor, St. Peterburg, FL	0.86
Tact	Hoya, Bethel, CT	Includes distance power
Technica	American Optical, Southbridge, MA	Includes distance power
Office	Shamir, San Diego, CA	0.75, 1.25, 1.75

designs with more than one power degression, the manufacturer has provided the laboratory with a selection guide based on the add power in the prescription (i.e., lower degressions are recommended with lower add powers). However, the practitioner can also specify the power degression in the prescription. This gives the practitioner considerable flexibility in designing the appropriate power in the top and bottom of the lens, dependent on the needs of the patient. This allows the practitioner to consider unique computer viewing distances or visual needs of the patient. For example, some patients sit almost continuously at their computer workstations, and far-intermediate vision in the top of the lens is unimportant. A lower degression would be suitable in this situation. A higher degression is indicated for the patient who regularly navigates the office and has extensive far-intermediate visual needs.

The following can be very effective at determining the most appropriate occupational progressive for a particular patient:

1. Measure the distance prescription and near (40 cm) add as usual. For example, +1.00 − 0.50 × 90, +2.00 add for OU.

2. In free space within your office, determine how much plus (in addition to the distance prescription) the patient will accept in the top of the lens. For this purpose, the patient should view objects at a distance that mimics his or her office setting. Lighting should be similar to typical office levels. Absolute clarity is not necessary; determine the level of blur, if any, the patient can accept in the top of the occupational progressive. This demonstration and measurement can usually be made with lens flippers over the patient's distance prescription. In this example, the patient accepts +0.75 for viewing at typical office distances.

3. The desired power degression in an occupational PAL is the difference between the near add and the acceptable plus determined above. In this example, the desired power degression is 1.25 D (2.00 − 0.75).

4. Select an occupational progressive design that provides the desired power degression. Write the prescription as follows:

OU +1.00 − 0.50 × 90, +2.00 add, Shamir Office, 1.25 degression.

The Technica lens (American Optical, Southbridge, MA) is prescribed in the same manner as a regular PAL prescription (i.e., prescribe the distance power along with the near add and place the fitting center at the pupil of the eye). The lens is designed to optimize the size of the lens area devoted to the intermediate powers. There is a large usable near area. The area of the lens devoted to the distance prescription is small and located near the top of the lens.

Occupational progressive lenses can very successfully meet the needs of most presbyopic computer users—subject to the same considerations given to fitting PALs for general wear. A favorable consideration is whether the patient is wearing PALs for general wear. Patients must be counseled that these lenses are specifically designed for use at the computer and that they should not be worn for other tasks, especially driving.

Optical contour plots of the major occupational lenses are shown in Figures 6-1 to 6-11. These measurements can be useful in helping to identify the lens design that will best meet the needs of your patient.

Bifocal Lenses

Flat top bifocals (usually FT28) with a computer prescription can work well for the more advanced presbyope for whom a single vision prescrip-

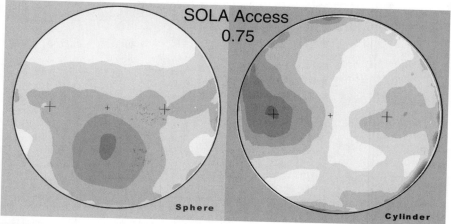

FIGURE 6-1. Access 0.75 (SOLA, Petaluma, CA). Contour plots (0.25 diopter steps) of spherical equivalent (0.00 to +1.00) and astigmatism (0.00–1.25). Measurements by COLTS Laboratory, Clearwater, FL.

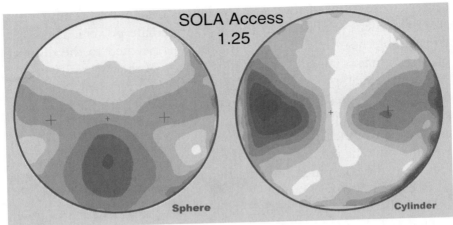

FIGURE 6-2. Access 1.25 (SOLA, Petaluma, CA). Contour plots (0.25 diopter steps) of spherical equivalent (–0.25 to +1.25) and astigmatism (0.00–1.75). Measurements by COLTS Laboratory, Clearwater, FL.

tion cannot meet both the intermediate and near visual needs, especially for patients who wear flat top bifocals to meet their general visual needs. In this case, the top of the lens contains the intermediate prescription, and the bottom contains the near prescription. The distance blur through the top of the lens must still be demonstrated to the patient; the

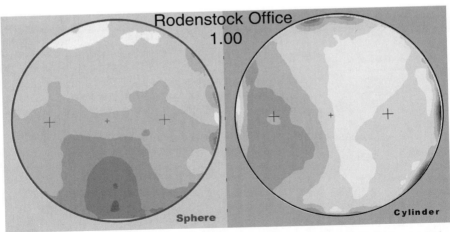

FIGURE 6-3. Cosmolit Office 1.00 (Rodenstock, Columbus, OH). Contour plots (0.25 diopter steps) of spherical equivalent (+0.25 to +1.50) and astigmatism (0.00–0.75). Measurements by COLTS Laboratory, Clearwater, FL.

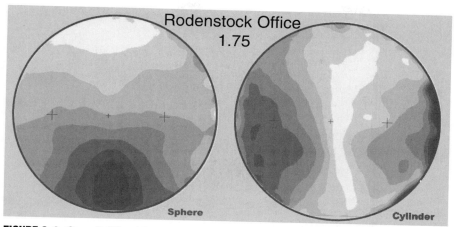

FIGURE 6-4. Cosmolit Office 1.75 (Rodenstock, Columbus, OH). Contour plots (0.25 diopter steps) of spherical equivalent (0.00 to +1.75) and astigmatism (0.00–1.50). Measurements by COLTS Laboratory, Clearwater, FL.

intermediate power can be trimmed a bit to lessen the distance blur. The prescription should be written with a note that it is for computer use, with the intermediate prescription as the main prescription and the add being the supplemental amount required to see at near. The bifocal can be fitted at the lower limbal margin as in most bifocal fittings.

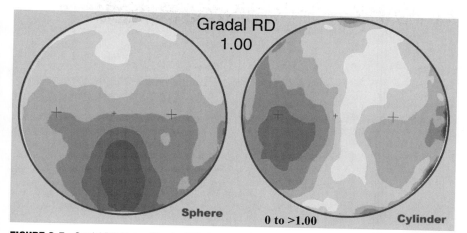

FIGURE 6-5. Gradal RD (Zeiss, Chester, VA). Contour plots (0.25 diopter steps) of spherical equivalent (+0.50 to +1.75) and astigmatism (0.00–1.00). Measurements by COLTS Laboratory, Clearwater, FL.

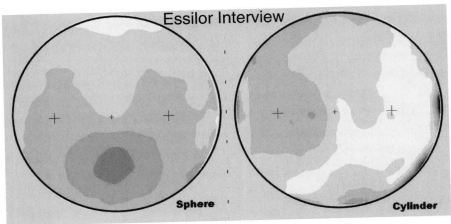

FIGURE 6-6. Interview (Essilor, St. Petersburg, FL). Contour plots (0.25 diopter steps) of spherical equivalent (+1.00 to +2.00) and astigmatism (0.00–0.75). Measurements by COLTS Laboratory, Clearwater, FL.

Less commonly, a bifocal lens can be prescribed for the person who needs only one lens power for the computer distance, but who is disturbed by the distance blur or has specific distance viewing requirements when working at the computer. In this case, the bifocal portion of the lens is used for the computer viewing, and it

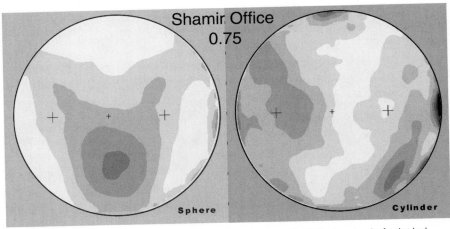

FIGURE 6-7. Office 0.75 (Shamir, San Diego, CA). Contour plots (0.25 diopter steps) of spherical equivalent (0.00 to +1.00) and astigmatism (0.00–1.00). Measurements by COLTS Laboratory, Clearwater, FL.

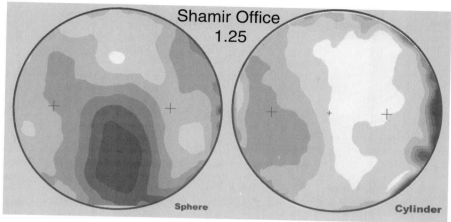

FIGURE 6-8. Office 1.25 (Shamir, San Diego, CA). Contour plots (0.25 diopter steps) of spherical equivalent (0.00 to +1.50) and astigmatism (0.00–0.75). Measurements by COLTS Laboratory, Clearwater, FL.

must be located appropriately. In nearly all cases, the bifocal needs to be fitted high, with the top of the segment located at mid-pupil or higher. The patient needs to be aware that the bifocal location makes it difficult to walk around the office and that the lens is not useful for meeting normal distance visual requirements. Another

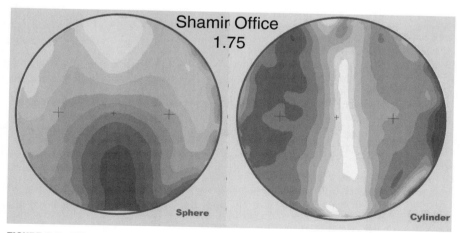

FIGURE 6-9. Office 1.75 (Shamir, San Diego, CA). Contour plots (0.25 diopter steps) of spherical equivalent (+0.25 to +2.50) and astigmatism (0.00–1.50). Measurements by COLTS Laboratory, Clearwater, FL.

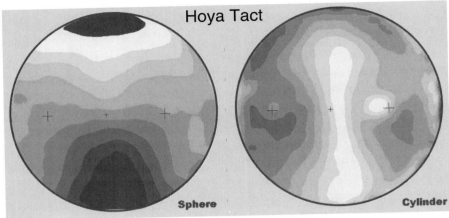

FIGURE 6-10. Tact (Hoya, Bethel, CT). Contour plots (0.25 diopter steps) of spherical equivalent (–0.25 to +2.00) and astigmatism (0.00–1.50). Measurements by COLTS Laboratory, Clearwater, FL.

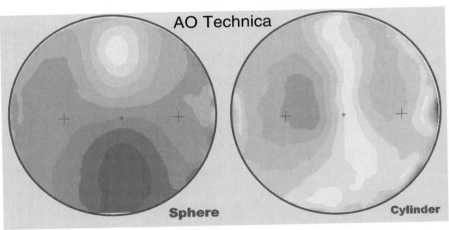

FIGURE 6-11. Technica (American Optical, Southbridge, MA). Contour plots (0.25 diopter steps) of spherical equivalent (0.00 to +2.00) and astigmatism (0.00–1.25). Measurements by COLTS Laboratory, Clearwater, FL.

strong consideration for this patient is the occupational progressive lens.

Trifocal Lenses

Trifocal lenses can be useful for the more advanced presbyopic patient who is intolerant of distance blur and requires clear distance vision while at his or her computer, and for whom occupational progressives are inappropriate (e.g., the patient uses bifocals or trifocals for general wear and is averse to progressives). Select a trifocal with a larger vertical dimension; they can be obtained with a 10-mm or 14-mm vertical size. The available occupational trifocal lenses are listed in Table 6-2. It is usually best to obtain a 60% intermediate add rather than the 50% add; this can be determined by measurement and demonstration as above.

Progressive Addition Lenses

Although PALs are very successful for general wear for many, if not most, patients, they often are not the best solution for a computer worker. This is because the width of the area of clear optics, especially that area of the lens containing the intermediate add needed for the

TABLE 6-2. Occupational trifocal lenses

Lens	Advantages	Disadvantages
X-Cel Acclaim 61	61% Intermediate segment; comes in 8 × 34, 10 × 35, 12 × 35	Appearance
SOLA E/D	Intermediate executive with 25-mm flat top bifocal	Executive ridge, weight, appearance
Vision-Ease FD	60% Intermediate	11-mm intermediate, appearance
Vision-Ease CRT DataLite	Large 14-mm intermediate	Executive ridges, weight, appearance
X-Cel CRT Trifocal	Same as above	Same as above

CRT = cathode ray tube.

computer working distance, is very narrow. This requires the patient to maintain a single fixed head position to see the screen clearly.

In some cases, the younger presbyope is able to successfully use PALs for computer work. Such a patient does not require the add for the intermediate viewing distance, something that can be determined in the demonstration process. The PAL can be successful in this case because the patient is able to use the distance portion of his or her lenses for work at the computer. The computer display should not be located too low on the patient's desk in this situation. The intermittent short-term computer user is another patient for which PALs are acceptable. In this situation, the work period is short and poor posture can be tolerated.

Conclusion

In most of the cases above, the prescription and spectacle design that best meet the visual needs at the computer are different than those required to meet the patient's other daily visual needs. This is likely to continue to be the case as long as we use computer monitors that are fixed to a desk surface and for which the users are required to orient themselves to the task rather than vice versa. Counseling is often necessary to demonstrate to patients that they require a separate pair of spectacles for their computer work.

Tints and Coatings

A pink tint can provide some symptom relief. Some patients who work in indoor environments, especially under fluorescent light, obtain increased comfort with light pink lenses. This obviously can apply to computer workers, because most offices are illuminated with fluorescent lights. The pink lenses serve to cut out some of the blue light emissions of the fluorescent lights, thereby decreasing the lights' brightness and decreasing fluorescence within the eye.

There is no specific need for ultraviolet (UV) protection at a computer. There is almost no UV emission from the computer or display. UV protection is certainly warranted for anyone exposed to significant

UV radiation, especially those who work in outdoor environments. However, there is no particular need for UV protection at a computer.

Antireflection coatings provide some benefit to those requiring spectacles at a computer workstation, as they similarly provide better vision in most environments. The antireflection coatings are on the surfaces of the spectacle lenses and significantly reduce reflections from the lenses. Light that is reflected from the back surface of the lens and then reflected again off the front surface ends up as improperly focused light that interferes with the primary image. For example, when looking into a dark café with a bright sky overhead, it is easier to see the detail in the dark café more clearly because light from the bright sky is not reflected inside the lens and hence on top of the image of the dark café. This can happen in a computer environment, especially one in which the screen has light characters on a dark background. Reflections from behind can be a source of annoying glare to a computer user, especially high myopes whose eyes are focused within 10 cm of the reflection. Antireflection coatings have increased value for patients with cataracts and macular degeneration who have decreased contrast sensitivity.

It is a common misperception that antireflection coatings on lenses reduce reflections off computer screens. This is because the reflections that occur on the video display terminal screen are well known, and, therefore, it is easy to assume that an antireflection coating on the spectacles improves the reflections in the screen. However, an antireflection coating on the spectacle lenses does not, in any way, reduce the reflection problems in the screen. Elimination of reflections off the computer screen are covered in Chapter 9.

Computer Glasses

Employers are increasingly finding it beneficial to provide computer glasses to their computer-using employees. This improves performance and comfort as well as employee morale. Very often the employee requires glasses for general wear and, for reimbursement purposes, it can be important to determine whether the glasses that are being prescribed are specifically for computer-viewing needs or if the glasses are essentially the same as those that the patient requires for general viewing needs.

The American Optometric Association (1995) has established criteria to determine when a pair of glasses can be considered "computer glasses." In general, glasses or other therapeutic eye care services are considered to be computer related if

- The person would not require the use of glasses or other treatment for a less visually demanding job.
- The glasses required for work at the computer are different in prescription power or design from those that would be required to meet the other general daily vision needs of the individual.

The American Optometric Association's specific requirements for computer glasses depend on the diagnosis as follows.

Presbyopia

Glasses for the correction of presbyopia are considered to be computer related if they are of a prescription power or lens or frame design that is different from that required for everyday visual needs. In general, this includes

- Single vision lenses prescribed specifically for the computer working distance
- Intermediate or near bifocals prescribed for use at the computer workstation
- Other special multifocal lenses prescribed for use at the computer workstation

Computer-related glasses would not include general-purpose single vision or multifocal lenses prescribed for everyday wear or PALs, except those designed specifically for computer operators.

Hyperopia

Glasses for the correction of hyperopia (farsightedness) are considered to be computer related if the individual would not otherwise require correction of his or her hyperopia for everyday visual needs.

Myopia

Glasses for the full correction of myopia (nearsightedness) are generally not considered to be computer related.

Astigmatism

Because of the visual demands of computer work, individuals with low amounts of astigmatism may require correction for computer tasks. Glasses are considered to be computer related if the individual would not otherwise require correction of astigmatism for general vision needs.

Glasses would generally not be considered computer related if the individual has moderate to large amounts of astigmatism (generally 1.00 D or greater), which require correction for habitual wear.

Heterophoria

Glasses that are prescribed for the correction of a clinically significant near heterophoria causing computer-related symptoms are considered to be computer related.

Convergence Insufficiency

A convergence insufficiency causing work-related symptoms is considered to be computer related. Vision therapy would be the treatment of choice for clinically significant convergence insufficiency.

Disorders of Accommodation

Treatment for disorders of accommodation causing work-related symptoms are considered computer related.

Glasses may be provided for the correction of clinically significant accommodative disorders in persons younger than 40 years.

Vision therapy for accommodative disorders may also be prescribed based on the judgment of the eye care provider.

Summary

Presbyopia offers many challenges to the clinician prescribing to maximize the comfort of his or her patients when using computers. New lens designs are being developed to fit the specific needs of our presbyopic computer users. More and more organizations are recognizing the benefit of supporting the provision of computer-specific glasses for workers. Chapter 7 further discusses ocular pathology conditions that can affect computer vision comfort.

Action Items

1. Contact your laboratory and get information on the computer-specific lens designs that they carry.
2. Ask the laboratory for consumer materials such as brochures or fact sheets.
3. Train your staff about the lens designs you plan to prescribe (Appendix 6-1).
4. Prescribe the appropriate computer lens design for yourself and staff members to experience.
5. Train staff on demonstrating prescribed lens designs, materials, tints, and coatings.
6. Train staff on proper measurement and fitting of computer-specific lens designs.
7. Be prepared to identify when a pair of glasses meets the criteria to be computer-specific eyewear.

References

American Optometric Association. Criteria for Determining Whether the Need for Eyeglasses or Other Treatment Is Related to Computer Use. St. Louis, MO: AOA,1995.

Bachman WG. Computer-specific spectacle lens design preference of presbyopic operators. J Occup Med 1992;34(10):1023–1027.

Brischer C, Mebine B, Osias GA. Working with task-specific progressive lenses. Opt Prism March 1994;4–16.

Butzon SP, Eagels SR. Prescribing for the moderate-to-advanced ametropic presbyopic VDT user: a comparison of the Technica and Datalite CRT trifocal. J Am Optom Assoc 1997;68:495–502.

Hanks A, Kris M, Peachey G, Simon A. A clinical wearer study of the Sola Access lens. Clin Exp Optom 1996;79(2):67–73.

Appendix 6-1

Staff Training Exercise

Explain the advantages and benefits of the following:

- Occupational progressive lenses
- Progressive addition lenses (PALs)
- Computer trifocals
- Large segment bifocals
- Single vision lenses
- Antireflection coatings
- Tints

What are the disadvantages of each?

How will you demonstrate the above lens characteristics?

Answer the question, "Why do I need a separate pair of glasses for working at my computer?"

What would you prescribe to the following patients?

1. A 50-year-old patient enters with a history of cataracts, diabetic retinopathy affecting the macula, and glaucoma. His vision is 20/60 through $+4.00 - 1.00 \times 90$ in each eye. He uses computers all day in his job as chief executive officer of an investment firm. Your examination supports the present medical treatment he is receiving. You can improve his distance vision to 20/40 through an increase of $+0.75$ diopter (D) in each eye. What may you prescribe for computer use?

2. A 60-year-old patient enters with the complaint of blurred vision at intermediate distances. The patient is presently wearing a

straight top bifocal. You find no change in the patient's prescription of +1.50 − 0.50 × 90 +2.50 add 20/20 OU. What may you prescribe for computer use?

3. A 42-year-old patient enters with no complaints; he works 4 hours per day at a computer. You find an increase in refractive error of −0.25 sphere OU from the patient's habitual (PAL) of −2.00 − 1.25 × 90, +0.75 add, 20/20 OU. The patient wears the PAL all day at work. What will you prescribe for general wear and for wear at the computer?

4. A 48-year-old patient enters complaining of blurred vision across the room through her new single-vision glasses that she received 3 months earlier from a competitor. You find the refractive error is +1.00 − 0.50 × 90 OU with a +1.75 add needed for 20/20 at 40 cm. The patient's single-vision prescription is +2.75 spheres. Her computer is at 50 cm.

5. A 52-year-old patient works at a water treatment plant, transferring readings from gauges 3–4 ft away from his computer, which is at 50 cm. His refractive error is −2.50 − 0.75 × 180 20/20 OU with a +2.00 add to 20/20 at 40 cm. Occasionally, he must see a clock at 20 ft. He is presenting wearing PALs but complains of the narrow intermediate vision.

Answers to Appendix 6-1

1. His decreased visual acuity is going to require a closer working distance than normal on the computer. In all probability, he will not be required to see farther than 6–10 ft across the room from his computer, yet he will desire a large viewing area on the lens. In his position as a chief executive officer, he will be conscious of his image, which probably eliminates an executive bifocal or ST 35. He would likely benefit from occupational progressive lenses. These lenses provide a wider area and better focus for intermediate distances than typical progressive lenses, yet also allow the person to see far-intermediate distances through the top of the lenses. See Occupational Progressive Addition Lenses for examples.

2. This patient may benefit from occupational progressives, but, because the patient is currently wearing bifocals for general eye wear,

the patient will most likely benefit from either intermediate-near bifocals or occupational trifocals. The intermediate-near bifocals will work best if the person performs dedicated work at the computer; the trifocals will be indicated if the person requires some distance vision while at the computer.

3. Prescribe the new glasses if the patient appreciates the improved distance vision. Because the patient is a beginning presbyope and has no complaints at the computer workstation, the patient will likely continue to successfully wear the PALs in the office.

4. Occupational progressive lenses will enable her to have good correction of intermediate and near distances and also allow her to see clearly at far-intermediate distances in the office. In the examination, determine how much plus she is able to accept when viewing at typical office distances—this is best done in free space. If, for example, she is satisfied with +0.50 add in the top of the lens, then you should select an occupational progressive with a power degression of 1.25 D (her near add is +1.75; 1.75 − 0.50 = 1.25).

5. An occupational progressive with a small area of distance power would work for this patient. The American Optical Technica is designed to provide this. An alternative would be to use another occupational progressive with a large degression—the largest alternative has a degression of 1.75 D. To use this as an alternative, determine whether the +0.25 of distance blur will be acceptable to the patient.

7
Treating Ocular Pathologic Conditions That Affect Computer Vision

Dry Eyes

Computer users commonly experience symptoms related to dry eyes. These complaints can include irritated eyes, dry eyes, excessive tearing, burning eyes, itching eyes, and red eyes. Contact lens wearers also often experience problems with their contact lenses while working at a computer display that are related to dry eyes. Whether the lenses are hard, soft, or gas-permeable, adequate tear configuration and flow are required for proper function and comfort. In response to the dry eye and the ocular irritation, reflex tearing sometimes occurs and "floods" the eyes with tears. This is the same reflex that causes tearing when we cry or when a foreign particle gets into our eye. On occasion, a patient may complain of watery eyes when, in fact, the cause is dry eye. Lemp (1998) reported that 35% of the U.S. population has symptoms related to dry eye.

Glands in the lids and conjunctiva continuously secrete the fluids and materials that are required to form the three layers of the tears. The total tear thickness is only approximately 7 μm, or .007 mm (Bartlett and Jaanus, 1995). Normally, the tear layers completely cover the anterior surfaces of the eye. Tears are lost via two mechanisms—drainage through the lacrimal duct and evaporation. Regular blinking is necessary to properly re-form the tear layer on a regular basis.

There are several reasons why computer workers are at greater risk for experiencing dry eye: decreased blink rate, larger palpebral aperture, lower workplace humidity, and incomplete blink due to higher viewing angle. An important finding has been that blink rate is significantly reduced during computer work. Yaginuma et al. (1990) measured blink frequency and lacrimation with electrode and cotton-thread methods, respectively, on four computer workers and noted that the blink rate during computer work dropped significantly compared to pre- and postwork measurements. There was no significant change in lacrimation. Patel et al. (1991) measured blink rate by direct observation on a group of 16 subjects. The mean blink rate during conversation was 18.4 blinks per minute and during computer use it was 3.6—more than a fivefold decrease. They also measured the tear thinning time (TTT) before and after computer work by observation of the time for keratometric mires to become distorted with the eye held open. The TTTs before and after computer use on the group of subjects were nearly identical, indicating no effect of video display terminal use on the TTT. Tsubota and Nakamori (1993) measured the blink rates of 104 office workers. The mean blink rates were 22 blinks per minute under relaxed conditions, 10 blinks per minute while reading a book on the table, and 7 blinks per minute while viewing text on a computer display. The data support the fact that blink rate decreases during computer use but also show that other tasks can decrease the blink rate. Possible explanations for the decreased blink rate include concentration on the task or a relatively limited range of eye movements.

Although book reading and computer work result in significantly decreased blink rates, computer work usually requires a higher gaze angle, resulting in an increased rate of tear evaporation. Tsubota and Nakamori measured a mean exposed ocular surface of 2.2 cm^2 while subjects were relaxed, 1.2 cm^2 while reading a book on the table, and 2.3 cm^2 while working at a computer. The size of the ocular aperture is related to the gaze elevation—as we gaze higher, our eyes are wider open. Because the primary route of tear elimination is through evaporation and the amount of evaporation is roughly linear with ocular aperture area, the higher gaze angle when viewing a computer display results in faster tear loss. Although reading a book and computer work both reduce the blink rate, the computer worker is more at risk because of the higher gaze angle.

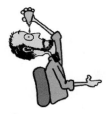

The most common clinical assessment of tear stability is probably evaluation of the tear breakup time (TBUT). This test is performed by instilling fluorescein in the tears (so that they can be seen with a slit lamp), holding the lids open, and then recording the length of time until the tears break up and expose the dry cornea. Normal individuals have a TBUT of 25–35 seconds, with a range of 15–45 seconds. Breakup times of less than 10 seconds are considered to be clinically significant. Individuals with marginal TBUT are at greater risk for having dry eye symptoms.

Franck (1986) found a statistically significant correlation between TBUT and eye irritation symptoms for 236 indoor office workers. Patel et al. (1991) argue that the TTT is a more valid measure because fluorescein can affect the tear stability. They cite data to show that a TTT of less than 12 seconds is clinically significant. It is reasonable to assume that tear film breakup results in drying of the ocular surfaces and that such drying results in surface irritation and symptoms. We can conclude that it is not good for the tear film to break up during the day.

There are many individuals with marginal TBUTs who do not have ocular drying with "normal" blink rates, but who do have regular ocular drying while working at a computer. With blink rates of approximately 20 blinks per minute, such as are measured during non-computer activities, ocular drying does not occur unless the TBUT is less than 3 seconds. However, for blink rates of 3.6 or 7.0 blinks per minute at computer work (as found in the studies), ocular drying occurs with a TBUT under 16.7 or 8.6 seconds, respectively. The decreased blink rate and increased rate of tear evaporation that occur with most computer work serve to put many workers over the edge; they experience ocular drying at the computer, although they do not experience it with other tasks.

There are other factors that may also contribute to the dry eye. For example, the office air environment is often low in humidity and can contain contaminants—there is extensive literature on sick building syndrome. It is also likely that the higher gaze angle results in a greater percentage of blinks that are incomplete. It is likely that incomplete blinks "don't count." This is because tear lipids normally pool along the lower lid margin, and during a full blink the upper eyelid grabs

---

Box 7-1

Ocular diseases that may contribute to dry eye symptoms
- Meibomian gland dysfunction
- Blepharitis
- Allergic conjunctivitis
- Blepharochalasis
- Trichiasis
- Lid abnormalities

---

the lipids and spreads them over the aqueous tear layer to form the lipid or oily layer of the tears. An incomplete blink does not allow this to occur; therefore, the evaporation-retarding properties of the lipid layer are lost.

Ocular disease (Box 7-1), allergic conjunctivitis, blepharitis, lid conditions, medications, natural aging, hormonal deficits as in menopause, and systemic disease (Box 7-2) may contribute to dry eye. Allergic conjunctivitis can result in papillae; blepharitis often is caused by staphylococcus bacteria, which release toxins into the eye at night, or scaling,

---

Box 7-2

Systemic diseases that contribute to dry eye
- Immunosuppressive diseases
- Lupus
- Thyroid disease
- Rheumatoid arthritis
- Diabetes
- Hormonal fluctuations
- Acne rosacea

Box 7-3

Medications contributing to dry eye

- Antihistamines
- Antihypertensives
- Anticholinergics
- Antidepressants
- Oral contraceptives
- Glaucoma medications
- Chronic medications with preservatives

which irritates the eye and causes dry eye. Lid abnormalities such as ectropion can cause an inability of the lids to properly spread the tears across the cornea epithelium. Medications like antihistamines, oral contraceptives, and antidepressants can lead to dry eye (Box 7-3). Oral skin condition medications such as isotretinoin (Accutane) can affect the oily layer, resulting in rapid evaporation of the tears. Keratoconjunctivitis sicca is commonly associated with arthritis or Sjögren's syndrome, which can have severe consequences and make computer work difficult. Ocular surface disease commonly accompanies dry eye. You can perform a dye test to confirm a dry eye diagnosis or to detect ocular surface disease (Karpecki and Thimons, 2001). Instill lissamine green or rose bengal dye (remember to administer an anesthetic drop before using rose bengal, because the dye stings). Look for staining of the nasal bulbar conjunctiva and staining along the top edge of the palpebral conjunctiva of the lower lid.

Staining indicates that ocular surface disease is present. Most such cases are secondary to keratoconjunctivitis sicca.

Laser in situ keratomileusis surgery can interrupt the neural feedback loop, which stimulates normal tear secretion. It generally takes 4–8 weeks for restoration of the neural feedback loop (Morris, 2000). Another theory is that the suction ring used during laser in situ keratomileusis surgery disrupts the high concentration of goblet cells at the limbus, decreasing mucin production.

Management

The data clearly show the reasons for dry eye difficulties for computer workers. The higher view angle results in faster tear evaporation. Also, the blink rate is significantly decreased. This is further compounded if the office environment is low in humidity. It has been shown that dry environments, such as on aircraft, result in complaints of dry eyes (Eng, 1979). There are many individuals with marginal dry eyes who do not experience symptoms in most environments, but who experience dry eye symptoms when working at a computer.

Management of the dry eye problem should include clinical treatment of the condition as well as consultation about working habits and the work environment. Contributing pathologic conditions are managed, accompanied by artificial tears or punctal plugs.

Step 1—Consider the ergonomics of the workstation. The computer screen should be placed so that the worker is habitually looking downward 10–15 degrees; usually, the top of the screen should be below eye level. Many workers, especially those who are shorter, are looking straight ahead or up at the computer display. In some cases, the computer display can be lowered by taking it off the central processing unit. If the patient works in a location with a ventilation breeze, he or she should change the airflow pattern or reorient the workstation. The patient should also be taught to blink more frequently, especially when he or she begins to notice the symptoms of dry eye. It helps to take an occasional 2-minute break, look into the distance, and concentrate on blinking.

Step 2—Educate your patients that their condition is chronic and may have many additional contributing factors (Karpecki and Thimons, 2001).

Step 3—Try to reduce the effect of these factors. For example, counsel patients to quit smoking, decrease caffeine intake, increase the amount of water they drink, and, perhaps, use a humidifier.

Step 4—The patient's prescribing physician may need to be consulted regarding changes in medication that could be aggravating the dry eye symptoms.

Step 5—Treat any complicating ocular conditions such as blepharitis, meibomianitis, or systemic causes. Blepharitis can be treated with lid scrubs or antibiotics, or both. Meibomianitis is treated with hot compresses for 10 minutes a day and with lid hygiene. Oral tetracyclines relieve severe blepharitis and meibomianitis as well as acne rosacea. Allergic conjunctivitis is often controlled with olopatadine (Patanol), ketotifen (Zaditor), or azelastine (Optivar), one drop b.i.d.

Cyclosporine A is an immunomodulatory drug that has significantly reduced symptoms of dry eye in clinical trials. Cyclosporine A inhibits the breakdown of the lacrimal and ocular surface. Dry eye may not only be caused by lack of tear production but also by a localized, immune-mediated inflammatory response affecting the lacrimal gland and ocular surface. Cyclosporine A is not yet approved for human use but is approved for veterinary use.

Step 6—Use ocular lubricants. Because preservatives can cause irritation, it is best to use preservative-free lubricants. An example may be one drop every hour.

A commonly used eye drop to replenish the mucous layer of tears is Viva-Drops (VISION Pharmaceuticals, Mitchell, SD). It is preservative-free and composed of a combination of antioxidants, a chelating agent, and a demulcent. Many patients prefer this lubricating drop.

A homeopathic drop used by many for comfort is Similisan No. 3 (Similisan Homeopathics, Fresno, CA). The company promotes the preservative-free drop as providing relief for computer vision syndrome. Many patients remark on how comfortable the drop is immediately upon instillation as compared to other tear supplements they have used in the past. Some patients prefer the homeopathic theory that Similisan No. 3 stimulates the eye's natural ability to relieve eyestrain due to intense computer work.

GenTeal (Novartis Ophthalmics, Duluth, GA) and Refresh Tears (Allergan, Irvine, CA) use a transiently preserved chemical that interacts with light to neutralize the preservative; therefore, there is no preservative toxicity. This is dependent on tears being present, so patients with extreme dry eye may be better off with preservative-free drops such as TheraTears (Advanced Vision Research, Woburn, MA), Celluvisc (Allergan, Irvine, CA), and Bion Tears (Alcon, Fort Worth, TX).

Step 7—Consider punctal occlusion to keep a sufficient reservoir of tears. Use dissolvable collagen implants as a diagnostic test. Insert the plugs into the inferior and superior canaliculi. Encourage the patient to use preservative-free artificial tears in conjunction with the implants. After a week, ask the patient whether the dry eye symptoms have improved. On occasion, the patient may experience itching in the inner corner of the lids. If so, the itching is most likely an indication that the patient is allergic to the collagen.

Contact Lens Wearers

Patients with dry eyes commonly benefit from wearing a low-water-content soft lens (AOA, 2000). Low-water-content lenses are best because they require less moisture from the eye to remain well hydrated. Daily-wear soft lenses also provide relief, particularly for patients experiencing allergies. The fresh soft lens avoids protein deposits on the front surface and may provide protection against airborne allergens. Hard, gas-permeable lens wearers often report relief from symptoms when switched to soft lenses. The availability of disposable soft trial lenses in astigmatic corrections facilitates the switch from gas-permeable lenses to soft lenses. If frequent prescription changes are anticipated, refit one eye at a time. Blink training can be especially beneficial to contact lens–wearing computer users. One of the best ways to treat dry eye patients who wear contact lenses is with punctal occlusion.

Cataracts

The clouding of the lens inside the eye results in increased haziness, causing blurred or distorted vision. Colors may seem yellowed and less vibrant. As cataracts progress, there is an increasing need for more light to see clearly. Lens distortion may cause double vision in one eye. All these effects on vision cause the computer user to have difficulties leading to symptoms when using the computer. Glare can be debilitating, and discriminating between the numbers 3, 5, and 8 may be difficult. The 3× rule discussed in Chapter 4 becomes significant to these patients. Antireflection coatings on computer glasses can help to improve contrast. Some patients experience more comfort by using Corning GlareControl lenses (Dow Corning Medical Optics,

Corning, NY). These are usually used when cataracts are accompanied by macular degeneration or diabetic retinopathy.

Macular Degeneration

A leading cause of vision loss among people over age 50 years, macular degeneration results in poor light adaptation, gradual loss of central vision, distorted vision, and decreased color vision. Vision at a computer often requires fixations from bright backgrounds to darker backgrounds. Patients with macular degeneration often have problems adapting to these changes in illumination; therefore, it is particularly important to have good lighting, as discussed in Chapter 8. The decreased visual acuity requires the 3× rule to be strongly considered. See Chapter 13 for details about managing low vision patients who work at computers.

Glaucoma

As the visual field diminishes, the glaucoma patient may be better off with a smaller character size to provide a bigger field of view. Glaucoma is one disorder in which the 3× rule may not be effective at providing comfort to the computer user. Other patients experiencing peripheral visual field loss, as in retinitis pigmentosa, may also be better off with smaller character size to allow use of the remaining central field to see words in the periphery.

Uncontrolled Diabetes

Patients with uncontrolled diabetes and fluctuating glucose levels may experience frequent refractive error changes. In the past, the changing refractive error could make it very difficult for a computer user to constantly change working distance and maintain the proper ergonomics necessary for comfort. Variable focus lenses and progressive addition lenses solve this problem to some extent. The computer user may have to adjust his or her head-tilt, but somewhere on the lens there is usually some usable vision to allow the patient to continue using his or her computer.

Corneal Dystrophies and Degeneration

Loss of transparency of the cornea results in light scatter and loss of contrast, which can make computer displays difficult to see. Antireflection coatings on their spectacles enhance contrast and improve vision. Often, patients with corneal dystrophies and degeneration respond well to tints blocking the short wavelengths of light, such as pink or rose tints. Specular reflections and office lighting can worsen the effects of corneal conditions.

Summary

Dry eye, ocular and systemic conditions, and computer vision symptoms can be exacerbated by environmental conditions present in the workstation. Lighting, reflections, computer displays, workstation ergonomics, and air quality can contribute to a worsening of symptoms. The following four chapters deal with environmental factors contributing to computer vision discomfort.

Action Items

1. Decide on a treatment regimen to alleviate dry eye symptoms.
2. Train staff to answer questions concerning dry eye and educate the computer user about contributing factors.
3. Obtain artificial tear samples and promotional materials.
4. Decide on which low-water-content contact lenses you will prescribe for contact-lens patients with dry eye.
5. Train staff to explain how ocular diseases can interfere with computer use.
6. Develop protocol for demonstrating antireflective coatings, tints, and Corning photochromic filter lenses to these patients.
7. Train your staff to explain workstation factors that may contribute to dry eye.
8. Create a handout to give to patients to self-evaluate their workstations.

References

AOA Optometric Clinical Practice Guideline: Care of the Contact Lens Patient. St. Louis: American Optometric Association, 2000.

Eng WG. Survey on eye comfort in aircraft: flight attendants. Aviat Space Environ Med 1979;50(4):401–404.

Franck C. Eye symptoms and signs in buildings with indoor climate problems. Acta Ophthalmol (Copenh) 1986;64:306–311.

Bartlett JD, Jaanus SD. Clinical Ocular Pharmacology, 3rd ed. Boston: Butterworth–Heinemann, 1995;256.

Karpecki PM, Thimons JJ. Dry eye management for the new century. Rev Optom 2001;138(2):64–72.

Lemp MA. Epidemiology and classification of dry eye. Adv Exp Med Biol 1998;438: 791–803.

Morris S. Postsurgical dry eye. Optom Manage May 2000;109–112.

Patel S, Henderson R, Bradley L, et al. Effect of visual display unit use on blink rate and tear stability. Optom Vis Sci 1991;68(11):888–892.

Tsubota K, Nakamori K. Dry eyes and video display terminals. Letter to editor. N Engl J Med 1993;328:524.

Yaginuma Y, Yamada H, Nagai H. Study of the relationship between lacrimation and blink in VDT work. Ergonomics 1990;33(6):799–809.

8
Lighting

There are several aspects of working at a computer that make it especially visually demanding or contribute directly to symptoms for computer users, or both. Mitigation of these problems can often directly eliminate symptoms or reduce the demands of the task so that symptoms don't result from marginal visual disorders. The most important visual environmental factors are listed in Box 8-1. They are presented in detail in this chapter, as well as Chapters 9–11.

General

Improper lighting is likely the largest environmental factor contributing to visual discomfort. Good lighting is actually quite easy to understand, but most people have a misconception concerning what is important about lighting. The common thought is that good lighting is evaluated on the basis of how much light is present, or the foot-candles (fc) of illumination. Although it is necessary and important to have adequate illumination, this is not usually the most important aspect of good lighting. In fact, there is often too much light in the office environment. The most important aspect of lighting is the distribution of light in the room.

The eye care practitioner's responsibility is to educate the patient on the effect of poor lighting on performance at the computer and to advise ways of improving the patient's situation. The eye care practitioner who offers site-visit evaluation of working environments can do lighting measurements and give proper recommendations.

Box 8-1

Aspects of the computer work environment that contribute to eye problems

- Lighting geometry and quantity
- Glare from windows or overhead lights
- Screen reflections
- Computer display design (contrast polarity, resolution, flicker, etc.)
- Workstation arrangement
- Office air quality

Making Light Measurements

Before having a discussion on light analysis, a few words on light measurements, the tools required for light measurements, and how to use the tools are required. There are two types of light measures that are critical in evaluating an office environment: illumination and luminance. Measuring these aspects of lighting can be very useful when performing on-site evaluations of a computer workplace (see Chapter 12).

Illumination is a measure of the amount of light (lumens) falling on a surface. The common units of illumination are fc (1 lumen/ft² of surface) and lux (1 lumen/m² of surface). There are 10.76 ft² contained within 1 m²; therefore, 10.76 lux is the same amount of illumination as 1 fc (i.e., the same light density per area). Lighting engineers and architects usually design the lighting in a room to provide a predetermined illumination level. An illumination meter is often simply called a *light meter* (Figure 8-1). The sensing device is simply placed at the location at which a measure of illumination is desired. Sometimes the sensing device is an integral part of the unit and sometimes extends from the unit with a wire attachment. Take care not to cast shadows on the measurement device while making a measurement. The measure of illumination depends on the height in the room—for example, it is typically

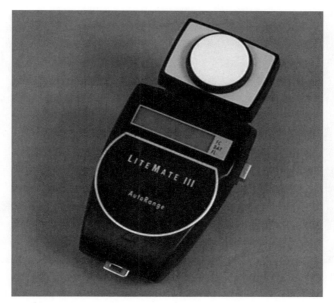

FIGURE 8-1. Example of a light meter that measures illumination.

greater at desk level than on the floor because of distance to ceiling lights. Normally, the illumination is measured on horizontal surfaces; therefore, the measuring device should be oriented horizontally. However, if you desire to measure illumination on the surface of the computer display, then the measuring device should be oriented parallel to the display surface. Illumination can vary quite widely in various office locations; therefore, it is important to measure it at the most important user locations and to specify where each measurement is made. For example, "General room illumination at desk level was 50 fc; at desks by the windows, it was 120 fc; and for those employees using a desk lamp, the reference materials had 90 fc of illumination."

Luminance is the other important measure of light. Luminance is the most important attribute insofar as vision is concerned, because it is a measure of the amount of light coming toward the eye from an object (per angular area of the object). Quite simply, we judge the brightness of objects based on their luminance. Brighter objects have higher luminance. The relationship between luminance and brightness is not

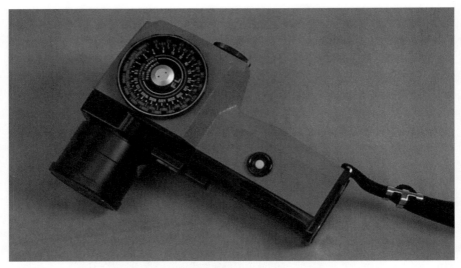

FIGURE 8-2. Example of a light meter that measures luminance.

linear—that is, each subsequent "step" in perceptual brightness requires a greater amount of luminance addition than did the previous step. This is similar to most other human senses such as sound and touch. The result of this nonlinear scaling is that our visual system is good at determining whether one object is brighter or dimmer than another, but our visual system is not good at judging the amount of luminance. This amount must be measured with a luminance meter or photometer (Figure 8-2). The common unit of luminance is candle/m² (cd/m^2).

The luminance of an object is measured by viewing it through a luminance meter. The viewer usually sees a circular reticle; the meter should be rotated so that this "measuring circle" is located on the object for which the luminance measurement is desired. (Most 35-mm cameras effectively measure luminance—that is, the user views the scene through the camera. The light needle moves or the camera settings change depending on the luminance of the scene.) For a valid measurement, the entire measuring circle should be filled with the object being measured. The same object can have a different luminance depending on the angle from which it is viewed. For example, the luminance (or brightness) of metal or glossy paper sitting on a table can change quite significantly if viewed from a different angle. Therefore, in computer-using environments, it is usually most important to make measurements from the normal location of the eyes of the computer user. Normally it is best to sit in the chair of the computer user to make the luminance measurements. A typical set of luminance measurements for a computer user might be

Computer display = 80 cd/m²
Reference documents = 150 cd/m² at 30 degrees to the left
Immediate background of display under shelving = 15 cd/m²
Open window in afternoon = 2,000 cd/m² at 50 degrees to the right
Overhead fluorescent lights = 3,000 cd/m²

Insofar as the visual system is concerned, luminance distribution in the field of view is the most important aspect of lighting. The geometry of the lighting in the room is normally the most important aspect of lighting as it relates to visual comfort. The geometry of the lighting is akin to the quality of the lighting. This involves not only the light sources, but also how the light is directed into the office through the use of lighting fixtures, baffles, blinds, drapes, and others and how it is reflected from the various surfaces in the room such as walls, ceilings, and furniture. A good lighting situation is one in which all of the visual objects in the field of view have nearly equal brightness (i.e., they all are similar in luminance). The correlate is that bad lighting is a situation in which objects in the field of view have large differences in luminance.

The most important principle of good lighting is to eliminate bright sources of light from the field of view and to obtain a relatively even distribution of luminance (brightness) in the field of view.

Glare Discomfort

Bright sources of light in the field of view create glare discomfort. Although this is a well-known phenomenon and the threshold sizes and locations of visual stimuli, which cause glare discomfort have been determined (Guth, 1981), the physiologic basis for glare discomfort is not known. It may be related to pupillary fluctuations. Because large brightness, or luminance, disparities in the field of view can cause glare discomfort, it is best to have a visual environment in which the luminances are relatively equal.

Primarily because of glare discomfort, the Illuminating Engineering Society (IES) has established and the American National Standards Institute (ANSI) has accepted (ANSI/IESNA, RP-1-1993) certain maximum luminance ratios that should not be exceeded. The luminance ratio should not exceed 1 to 3 or 3 to 1 between the task and the immediate visual surroundings (approximately 25 degrees), nor should the ratio exceed 1 to 10 or 10 to 1 between the task and more remote visual surroundings (ANSI/IESNA, RP-1-1993). A person is at greater risk for experiencing glare discomfort when the source has a higher luminance and when the source is closer to the fixation point (Box 8-2).

Box 8-2

Display and glare source luminance

Visual object	Luminance (candle/m^2)
Dark background display	20–25
Light background display	80–120
Reference material with 75 footcandles	200
Reference material with auxiliary light	400
Blue sky (window)	2,500
Concrete in sun (window)	6,000–12,000
Fluorescent lights (poor design)	1,000–5,000
Auxiliary lamp (direct)	1,500–10,000

There are many objects in the field of view that can cause luminance ratios in excess of those recommended by ANSI/IES. Box 8-2 lists the typical luminance of objects in the field of view. The luminance of the screen should be noted first, because it is the screen that the person is viewing. This usually sets the lower end of the luminance ratio. The luminance values in Box 8-2 readily show that luminance ratios can greatly exceed those recommended by ANSI/IES.

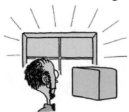

The glare sources are a particular problem for computer workers who are generally gazing horizontally in the room. This results in light fixtures and other glare sources being closer to the fixation point for today's computer worker compared to yesterday's office worker who looked down at the desk. Bright open windows pose the same risk as overhead light fixtures. Workers are also at greater risk for discomfort glare if they use a dark background computer display, resulting in greater luminance disparity between the task and other objects in the room. Other sources of large luminance at the computer workstation include white paper on the desk, white desktop surfaces, and desk lamps aimed toward the eyes or that illuminate the desk area too highly.

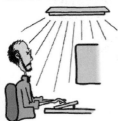

A common source of discomfort glare is shown to the left. Light often leaves the overhead fluorescent fixture in a wide angle, resulting in light directly entering the eyes of the workers. It is very common for the luminance of the fixture to be more than 100 times greater than that of the video display that the worker is viewing, far exceeding the IES recommended maximum.

Good lighting design can significantly reduce discomfort glare. Light leaving the fixture can be directed so that it goes straight down and not into the eyes of the room occupants. This is most commonly accomplished with the louvers in the luminaire or fixture. However, this results in severe shadows, and the glare is still there; it is just more peripheral in the field of view. An even better solution is indirect lighting in which the light is bounced off the ceiling, resulting in a large low-luminance source of light for the room.

Glare—Other Visual Problems

Another problem that occurs with large disparities in the brightness of objects in the field of view is that, when looking from brighter objects to darker objects or vice versa, there is always a brief period of time after the eye movement during which the eye has to adapt to the new brightness level. This is called *transient adaptation*. Entering or leaving a dark movie theater or restaurant in the daytime is a common example of dark and light adaptation. These are situations in which the eye needs to completely adapt to a different range of brightness. This same effect occurs on a smaller scale when the eye needs to fixate back and forth from bright to dark objects in a given environment. When the eye is not properly adapted to the brightness level at which it is looking, the vision is not good. This is a particular problem when constantly looking back and forth from a dark background computer display to a bright white reference document (see Box 8-2).

Patients who have macular degeneration are susceptible to symptoms caused by difficulties with light adaptation. The lower number of healthy cone photoreceptors requires a longer period to recover from being dazzled by glare. Consider this factor as a source of problems for older patients.

Illumination Levels

A goal of illuminating a computer work environment should be not to cause glare discomfort. Therefore, the 1 to 3 and 3 to 1 recommended maximum luminance ratios can be used to establish recommended illumination ranges based on ratios to the screen luminance. Because the computer display is the primary visual target, it is important to balance the luminance of the display with the lighting in the work environment. The luminance (brightness) of most objects that are visually adjacent to the computer are dependent on the amount of the room illumination and on the reflectance of each of those objects. Ideally, the luminance of the computer display is matched (within a factor of 3) with the general luminance of nearby objects in the environment. If this is not the case, then consider adjusting the display brightness or the room illumination to accomplish parity.

Is Glare Discomfort Present?

Subjective Method

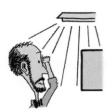

One way to test for glare discomfort is to have the worker look at his or her computer screen and be aware of any bright lights in the worker's peripheral vision. The worker can use his or her hand to shield the eyes like a baseball-cap visor and should note whether he or she senses an immediate improvement in comfort. If the glare is from the window, then shield the eyes from the window. The worker should try this two to three times. If he or she notices an immediate sense of improved comfort by eliminating the lights from peripheral vision, then the worker is experiencing glare discomfort. Most people, when performing this test in the presence of bright overhead fluo- rescent lights, notice the discomfort glare. If they can notice an immediate improvement in com- fort, the cumulative effects of an entire workday are quite obvious.

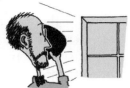

Measurement Method

A luminance meter can be used to measure the luminance of key objects in the field of view to determine whether they may cause glare discomfort. Measurements should be made with the instrument view- ing from approximately the same location as the user's eyes. It is best to use a fairly large aperture size (approximately 1 degree) so that the spatially averaged luminance value of a given stimulus can be deter- mined. The luminance levels of detail (e.g., the luminance of the text letters) are not important; rather, the mean luminance of large areas within the visual field is important. Typical measurements would be to measure the luminance level of the screen (large aperture to include text and screen background), the reference document, the wall or desk area behind the computer, general office luminance, desk lamp, window, and overhead lights. For each measurement, it is also important to note the angle between the normal line of sight to the computer and the line toward the glare source. This angle can be measured or estimated by viewing the computer user from the side and viewing the geometry through a clear protractor.

The luminance ratios of the peripheral objects to the computer display can then be determined and compared to the maximum recommended luminance ratios established by the IES. The luminance ratio should not exceed 1 to 3 or 3 to 1 between the task and the immediate visual surroundings (within 25 degrees), nor should the ratio exceed 1 to 10 or 10 to 1 between the task and more remote visual surroundings. The dividing angle of 25 degrees can be estimated as being 50% percent (actually 46.6%) of the distance from the eyes. For example, for a fixation point at a viewing distance of 24 in., an object that is 12 in. (11.2 in.) laterally from the fixation point would be 25 degrees away.

Clinical Method

Although there is not a clinical method for measuring discomfort glare (tests of disability glare do not test for glare discomfort), it is quite easy to demonstrate to patients as follows. In most eye care offices, there is an overhead fluorescent fixture that is quite bright. If this is not available, a bright open window or a desk lamp can also serve for the demonstration. Instruct the patient to look straight ahead at a fixation point with the bright light in his or her peripheral vision. Encourage the patient to continue viewing the fixation point while shielding and unshielding his or her eyes several times. If the patient notes glare discomfort, then advise the patient to perform the same test while looking at his or her computer. Positive results help the patient to identify sources of glare discomfort and, hence, what he or she should attempt to treat or eliminate in his or her work environment.

Solutions to Glare Discomfort

If bright lights are deemed to contribute to discomfort, then they should be removed or mitigated in some manner. There are several ways in which the situation can be improved. Many of the solutions below are suggestions that can be implemented fairly inexpensively by the computer user and without major office redesign.

1. Turn off the offending fluorescent lights. Sometimes, it is a single offending fluorescent fixture in the ceiling that is immediately in front of the person. The entire fixture can often be turned "off" by loosening one of the fluorescent tubes. Very often, a single offending fixture can be turned off without creating lighting deficiencies. Many offices have too much light anyway. When turning off lights, however, consideration must be given to coworkers, who may rely on the light coming from that particular fixture.

2. Many offices have two wall switches controlling the fluorescent light fixtures. Each switch controls half of the bulbs in all of the fixtures. Often, both switches are turned on for the day. If the room is brighter than the computer displays, consider turning off half of the lights. Very frequently, however, people are more comfortable with only one switch turned on, effectively cutting the room illumination in half. The first reaction of many people on turning off half of the lights is negative. However, request that they try it for a few minutes. After they have worked in the reduced illumination for a while, most people forget that the light level is lower and appreciate the improvement.

3. Some fluorescent light fixtures can be retrofitted with parabolic louvers that direct the light straight down into the room. The reason that fluorescent lights cause discomfort glare is that most of the light fixtures direct the light so that it leaves the fixture in all directions. This results in light leaving the fixture toward the eyes of workers who are looking horizontally in the room. A parabolic louver (the louver is the egg crate–like cover that directs light into the room) directs the light from the fluorescent tubes straight down; hence, the light is not directed into anyone's eyes.

4. Reorient the workstation so that bright lights are not in the field of view. Sometimes the work desk can be rotated 90 or 180 degrees so that the fluorescent lights or bright windows are not in the field of view. Many workers make the mistake of placing their computer display immediately in front of a window. In this situation, the brightness ratio between the screen and the window can be excessive. In a large office with rows of overhead fluorescent lights, it is usually better if workers look along the rows of lights while viewing the computer display instead of across the rows.

5. Wear a visor. This is actually a very efficient way to eliminate the brightness of overhead fixtures. A person can wear a visor for a day or two as a test to determine the extent to which the visor alleviates discomfort at the end of the day. This can help the worker and his or her manager or doctor gauge the 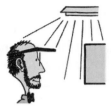 extent to which overhead brightness is contributing to the worker's discomfort and the extent to which solutions should be implemented.

6. Avoid bright reflective surfaces. In some work environments, the desktops are white. This is not good because it results in the desktop surface becoming a discomfort glare source. Desktops and other furnishings should have a matte, medium-reflective surface. Ceilings should be painted white, and walls should be medium light.

7. Use blinds or drapes on windows. This is often the most difficult change to implement because people like window views. However, if the window view is considerably brighter than objects in the room (as it normally is), then the window is serving as a discomfort glare source. Usually, the best solution is to use blinds. The blinds should be adjusted so that the worker cannot see the light coming from the window, but the light from the window should be directed upward onto the ceiling or sideways so that it is not entering the worker's eyes. (The light should also be directed so that it is not directly hitting the computer screen, which causes screen reflections.)

8. Evaluate whether auxiliary lighting (e.g., a desk lamp) on reference documents is causing glare discomfort. Auxiliary lighting is not often necessary and may contribute to glare discomfort. General room illumination is often adequate to see the reference documents clearly. Placing the auxiliary lighting on reference documents often causes them to become considerably brighter than the computer display, especially if it is a dark background display. The bright reference document not only creates a discomfort glare source, but it also results in transient adaptation problems when looking back and forth from the dark screen to the bright reference documents. The first impression on turning off auxiliary lighting is often negative; therefore, longer-term comfort should serve as the guide to changes.

9. Change the brightness of the screen. The brightness of the screen should be adjusted to match the brightness of the visual objects

that immediately surround it. This is usually accomplished quite easily with a display with black characters on a white background. It is not possible to accomplish this if the display has light characters on a dark background—the worker is looking into a "black hole" surrounded by a much brighter room. This results in a fundamentally poor visual environment and is one of the primary reasons why light background displays are preferred over dark background displays for most purposes.

10. Hang or erect partitions. Very often, the offending light sources can be eliminated from the field of view by erecting or moving partitions.

In summary, lighting is often the most significant factor in the work environment resulting in vision discomfort at the computer. Patients must be educated as to the effect of improper lighting and instructed on how to improve it. Appendix 8-1 shows a sample handout that may be given to patients to self-evaluate the lighting in their work area. Chapter 9 addresses a second major work environment factor, reflections.

References

ANSI/IESNA RP-1-1993. American National Standard Practice for Office Lighting. New York: American National Standards Institute, 1993.

Guth SK. Prentice Memorial Lecture: The science of seeing—a search for criteria. Am J Optom Physiol Opt 1981;58:870–885.

Appendix 8-1

Lighting at a Computer Workstation

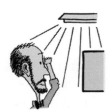 Although the amount of light is important, it is more important to have good light distribution. Good light distribution is accomplished when all of the objects in the field of view have approximately equal brightness. Bright lights or windows are common offending sources and cause discomfort. You can determine if the overhead lights or windows are contributing to discomfort by shielding them from the field of view with a hand or a file folder, which simulates a visor. If a small but immediate sense of relief occurs, the bright source is contributing to discomfort.

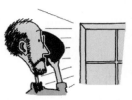

Suggestions for improving the lighting include the following:

1. Use blinds or drapes on windows to eliminate the bright light. It is often necessary to change the blind adjustment during the day because of sun movement. The blinds should be adjusted to allow light into the room without being able to see the bright light directly.
2. It is often inadvisable to put additional lighting on reference documents; this makes them too bright compared to the screen.
3. If auxiliary desk lighting is used, it should be low wattage and be directed so that it does not directly enter your eyes or directly illuminate the computer screen.
4. Indirect lighting systems often provide the best visual environment.
5. Wear a visor to shield your eyes from bright overhead lights.
6. Reorient the workstation so that bright lights are not in the field of view.

7. Avoid white reflective surfaces. Desktops and other furnishings should have a matte, medium-reflective surface.
8. Ceilings should be painted white, and walls should be medium light.
9. Turn off some fluorescent light fixtures that are in your field of view and are bothersome. Be considerate of the effects on other employees. More information is available at http://www.DoctorErgo.com.

9
Reflections from the Computer Display

The surface of a cathode ray tube (CRT) screen is glass and obviously reflects light. As discussed in Sources of Display Reflections, however, reflections from the phosphor coating on the inside of the glass are often more problematic than the reflection from the glass surface. Reflected light enters the eye along with the images being viewed on the screen. This results in a degradation of the visual image. Trying to read a degraded image can certainly contribute to eyestrain or other visual discomfort.

Reflected Light—Background

Reflections can be categorized as diffuse or specular. In reality, most surfaces have both a diffuse component and a specular component to their reflectance pattern. Matte surfaces have more diffuse reflectance, whereas shiny materials such as metal or glossy paper have a large specular component.

A perfectly diffuse reflector (sometimes called a *Lambertian surface*) is characterized by the fact that the portion of light reflected in any direction from the surface is independent of the direction from which the surface was illuminated. Another characteristic is that the amount of light reflected at any given angle (α) from the perpendicular is decreased by $\cos(\alpha)$. Because the projected image size (as viewed by the eye) of an object is also decreased by $\cos(\alpha)$, the light being received per unit projected area of the object remains the same (i.e., the retinal illumination is independent of viewing angle). The net result is that a diffuse reflector has the same luminance and, hence, appears to have the same brightness when viewed from any angle.

A specular reflector is one for which the amount of light reflected is highly dependent on the angle of the incident light and the direction in which the reflected light is measured. A perfect specular reflector would be a mirror in which all of the reflected light would obey the law of reflection—that is, the angle of reflection (measured from the perpendicular to the surface) is equal but opposite to the angle of the incident light. The luminance and, hence, the perceived brightness of a specular surface are highly dependent on the angle of incidence of the light and the angle from which the surface is viewed. Reading a glossy magazine surface becomes nearly impossible if the desk lamp is oriented so that the specular reflections enter the eyes; likewise, the reflection of a window on the glass surface of a CRT makes reading a computer monitor difficult.

Another distinction between specular and diffuse reflections concerns polarization. Diffuse reflections are never polarized, regardless of the polarized state of the incident light. Specular reflections, on the other hand, can be highly polarized depending on the polarization state and angle of incidence of the incoming light. For example, the primary effect of polarized sunglasses is to eliminate specular reflections from windows, metal, and water.

Sources of Display Reflections

CRT screens have a glass surface; therefore, most of the reflected light is specular and results in a "mirror-like" image of the light source. If the glass surface is frosted, this adds a diffuse component to the reflection from the glass. Although this reflection from the glass surface can be very bothersome and certainly noticeable, it is often not the most problematic reflection. Usually, the most problematic and insidious reflection is from the phosphor (the powder-like coating on the inner glass surface). The phosphor is the material that emits light when struck by the electron beam and is similar to the coating on the inside surface of a fluorescent light tube. Although phosphor glows when struck by an electron beam, it also passively reflects light similar to the way a sheet of paper does. Reflections from the phosphor are diffuse.

Turning off the computer is a good way to observe reflections. When the computer screen is off, the display is as black as anything on the screen ever gets! The lack of complete blackness is due to the diffuse reflections of general room light. Any specular reflections from the glass are seen as "hot spots" of reflected light in the screen.

Effects of Specular Reflections

Specular reflections from the glass surface of the CRT create images of the sources, often windows behind the user, that appear as hot spots of light in the screen and can make it impossible to see the screen image at the location of the specular reflection. This is bothersome at the least and prevents the person from seeing that part of the screen or causes them to move to see around the reflection. This can contribute to vision problems and to musculoskeletal stress. It has been often suggested that the images formed by specular reflections can interfere with the normal accommodative response to the display. However, Collins et al. (1994) determined that such reflections do not alter the accommodative response.

Effects of Diffuse Reflections

Because reflections from the phosphor in a CRT are diffuse, a portion of any light impinging on the screen, regardless of the direction from which it comes, is reflected into the eyes of the user and causes the screen to appear brighter. This means that black is no longer black, but a shade of gray. The diffuse reflections add equally to the luminance of the black and the white portions of the display and, hence, reduce contrast of text presented on the screen. Instead of viewing black characters on a white background, gray characters are presented on a white background. The reflections seem to cause more disruption with the opposite polarity (i.e., white characters on a black [gray] background). The decreased contrast makes it more difficult for the eyes to focus, maintain binocularity, and quickly and efficiently move over the text. Working under these conditions increases the demand on the visual system and can aggravate accommodative disorders, binocular dysfunction, and refractive disorders.

In the sample shown in Box 9-1, screen reflections reduce contrast from 96% to 53%.

Antireflection Screens or Filters

An antireflection (AR) filter placed over the computer display is the most common and often the most effective way to resolve diffuse reflection problems. The primary purpose is to decrease the luminance of "black" by an amount greater than "white," thereby increasing the contrast. Scullica et al. (1995) compiled symptom information on 25,064 workers, 28% of whom used AR filters. Scullica et al. did not measure a relationship between symptoms and use of an AR screen. However, Hladky and Prochazka (1998) used 60 subjects divided into a control group and a study group and determined that the group using the AR filters had fewer symptoms. In a laboratory study, Wacker et al. (1999) determined that reading and letter-counting performance are better with less reflected glare. The beneficial effects of AR filters on contrast in properly selected situations are certain. Use of AR filters in such situations can mitigate symptoms and improve performance, although using an AR filter is not a panacea.

Most AR screens today are glass or plastic. Mesh filters, not commonly used anymore, are comprised of black cloth material tightly drawn onto a frame that fits over the computer display. The principle of operation can be likened to a screen door—light impinging on the screen at an oblique angle is unable to pass through the filter. Likewise, the mesh filter in front of the computer screen blocks light that enters the screen obliquely, such as from fluorescent lights in the ceiling or windows on a side wall. If the light cannot get through to the screen, it does not come back out as a reflection. Mesh filters can be effective at making the screen blacker, and they have the advantage that they are usually less expensive than glass and plastic filters. However, mesh filters have the major drawback that they significantly reduce screen resolution because the user now views through a piece

Box 9-1

Sample calculation of the effects of diffuse reflections on contrast

- Formulae:

  Contrast $(C) = |(L_t - L_b)/(L_t + L_b)|$

  L_b = luminance of the background

  L_t = luminance of the target or characters

  The offending light source results in illumination (E) on the screen that, after reflectance (r is the diffuse reflectance factor of the screen) becomes reflected luminance. The formula for this process is $L = Er/\pi$.

  The conversion factor from the English unit of footcandle (fc) to the metric unit of candle (cd)/m² is 10.76.

- Sample:

  L_b is 100 cd/m² in a dark room (white background)

  L_t is 2 cd/m² in a dark room (black target or letter)

  Room illumination is 75 fc on a horizontal surface, therefore approximately 40 fc on the vertical screen.

  Screen reflectance is 30%.

  Calculated screen contrast in a dark room is

  $C = |(100 - 2)/(100 + 2)| = 0.96 = 96\%$

  Calculations of $L_t + L_b$ and contrast with room lights on

  $L_b = 100 + (40 \times 0.30 \times 10.76/\pi) = 141$ cd/m²

  $L_t = 2 + (40 \times 0.30 \times 10.76/\pi) = 43$ cd/m²

  $C = (141 - 43)/(141 + 43) = 0.53 = 53\%$

of cloth. Glass and plastic filters do not have this compromise and, hence, have largely displaced mesh filters.

Glass or plastic filters primarily act as a neutral density filter—the most common transmittance is 30%. Because reflected light must pass through the filter twice, the luminance of reflections is reduced more than tenfold (30% × 30% = 9%). The effect is to make "black" blacker by the square of the filter transmittance. This significantly improves the contrast yet, because the patient is viewing through a clear optical element, there is no significant loss in the resolution of the screen characters.

The primary purpose of glass and plastic AR screens is to make the blacks blacker, thereby increasing the contrast. The luminance of light that is emitted by the screen (the desired "white" image) is decreased by the transmittance factor of the filter, whereas light that is reflected from the computer screen (undesired light) is decreased by the square of the filter transmittance because it must pass through it twice. Because the luminance of the blacks (with room lights on and, therefore, in the presence of reflections) has a much greater percentage contribution from reflected light than do the whites, the blacks receive a greater percentage decrease in luminance than do the whites. A calculation of the effect of a glass AR filter on the contrast is shown in Box 9-2.

In the example, the contrast of 96% in a dark room is reduced to 53% because of reflections but improved to 77% with a 30% AR filter. If the screen brightness can be increased to help compensate for the filter, the contrast gains calculated in Box 9-2 are understated.

AR filters improve contrast, but they also decrease the screen luminance, thereby potentially causing the screen to become significantly darker than the surrounding visual stimuli and potentially violating the 1 to 3 luminance ratio recommendation for discomfort glare discussed in Chapter 8. The extent of this potential problem depends on the display polarity, the luminance adjustment range of the display, and the transmittance of the AR filter.

Screen reflections are particularly problematic if the person is using a dark background display (i.e., light characters on a darker background). Contrast reduction is particularly notable with this screen polarity. With a dark background display, it is likely that the screen luminance is already too dark compared to surrounding luminance. A

Box 9-2

Effect of antireflection filter on display contrast

Example:

Use the previous example (Box 9-1) in which contrast was 96% in a dark room and 53% with room lights.

Add a 30% transmittance glass antireflection filter.

Calculated screen contrast with room lights on and 30% filter

$$L_b = (100 \times 0.3) + (40 \times 0.30 \times 10.76/\pi)(0.09) = 33.7 \text{ candle (cd)/m}^2$$

$$L_t = (2.0 \times 0.3) + (40 \times 0.30 \times 10.76/\pi)(0.09) = 4.3 \text{ cd/m}^2$$

$$C = (33.7 - 4.3)/(33.7 + 4.3) = 0.77 = 77\%$$

---

first step would be to determine if the individual can switch polarity. If not, however, in this situation the loss in screen luminance by using an AR filter is probably small with respect to the very significant gain in contrast. An AR filter is especially indicated for a dark background display in the presence of screen reflections.

For white background screens, more care must be taken not to make the screen too dark compared to the environment. Depending on the brightness adjustment range of the computer display and on the room illumination, it may be possible to completely offset the loss of luminance of the whites caused by the filter by adjusting the screen brightness. However, some displays may not have enough adjustment range to compensate for the effects of the filter; this is often the case with older displays. In these situations, especially in the presence of bright office lighting and, hence, bright immediate surroundings, it is better to use a lighter AR filter (higher transmittance). Lighter AR filters do not reduce reflections as well, but they also do not decrease the screen luminance as much; they are indicated in brighter rooms with dimmer displays.

Glass and plastic filters must be AR coated so that the surfaces of the AR filter do not create reflection problems. Without a coating, a glass surface reflects approximately 4% of the incident light as a specular reflection. It is essential to put an AR coat on the front surface of the filter. Coating the back surface of the filter is desirable, but not as essential because the reflection from the back surface is reduced by the square of the filter transmittance. As with any optical coatings, it is important that they be kept clean for optimal performance.

Some glass or plastic filters have a circular polarized element in them. This feature results in circular polarized light being transmitted to the computer screen. The resulting specular reflection from the screen surface changes the rotation of the polarization of the light so that it is blocked from coming back out through the filter. Because only specular reflected light maintains its polarized properties after reflection, this polarizing feature provides added benefit only for specular reflections.

Some AR filters are classified as *privacy filters*. Such filters have microlouvers in them that prevent seeing the display from oblique angles. These filters are indicated for people who view sensitive documents and are often useful for air travelers.

Treating Reflection Problems

Are Reflections a Problem?

People are usually unaware of screen reflections because they are so intent on seeing the characters on the screen. An analogous situation is viewing merchandise through a display window. Most people are seldom aware of window reflections that degrade visibility of the merchandise. An amateur photographer can be tricked by these reflections and not notice them until the photograph is developed. Because people are seldom even aware of noticeable specular reflections and are much less likely to be aware of diffuse reflections, computer users need to be given observation tools to evaluate whether bothersome reflections exist.

Specular reflections are best observed with the computer display turned off or with a dark background on the display. Observe any specular reflections and identify their source. Then turn the screen back on. If the reflections are still noticeable and interfere with the visibility of the characters on the screen, then the reflections are causing difficulties and should be addressed.

Diffuse reflections can be identified by using file folders as temporary hand-held light baffles to block room light from illuminating the computer screen. Identify the major directions from which light is impinging the screen and use the folders to block all such light. For example, for light coming from the ceiling, place the folder as if placing a visor on the computer; if the offending light source is a window on the side of the display, then place the light baffle on the side of the computer display. Look at the screen images with and without the baffle(s) in place and note whether the baffle improves the contrast and clarity of the images on the screen. If there is a noticeable improvement in the image quality on the screen, then diffuse reflections are a problem and should be addressed.

Workstation Changes

The first step, especially for specular reflections, is to determine whether the source of the reflections can be removed. This can often be done by using blinds or drapes on windows, turning off a light fixture in the ceiling, etc. It is usually not possible to eliminate fully screen reflections by controlling the sources, but the reflections may be reduced to more acceptable levels.

Also consider changing the tilt or swivel position of the display within acceptable ergonomic limits; this can be particularly effective at eliminating specular reflections. Rearranging the workstation can also eliminate specular reflections.

Antireflection Filters

AR filters that fit over the computer display are the most common and often the most effective way to solve reflection problems, especially diffuse reflections.

Mesh AR filters are not as effective as glass or plastic AR filters and are not used much any more. They operate similar to a screen door by blocking light from oblique angles. They are relatively inexpensive, but their major drawback is that viewing the screen through the mesh reduces resolution.

Glass or plastic AR filters are a more effective option because they do not significantly degrade the image on the computer display. However, the glass and plastic AR filters are more costly because of the more expensive material and because of the AR coating that must be placed on the glass. Also, the coating is very sensitive to dirt and fingerprints; some effort is required to keep the screen clean.

An AR filter reduces screen luminance, and this must be considered in selecting a filter. It is important that the display not become too dark compared to adjacent visual objects. If the maximum display brightness is quite high, especially 100 candles (cd)/m^2 or better, then a typical AR filter with approximately 30% transmittance will work well. It is likely that the screen will still be bright enough with the filter in place to stay within lighting guidelines as discussed in Chapter 8. If, however, the screen is not very bright (especially if the maximum luminance is 50 cd/m^2 or less), then a lighter AR filter with greater transmittance should be obtained. A lighter AR filter is not as effective at reducing reflections. If the computer screen is not very bright, consider replacing it.

If significant specular reflections are present and cannot be resolved by eliminating the source or adjusting the position of the display, an AR filter with circular polarization is indicated.

The American Optometric Association (AOA) has established minimum quality specifications for AR filters. Manufacturers who can show compliance with the AOA specifications are able to have their product accepted by the AOA and to use this fact in product promotion. This has become a de facto standard, and most major manufacturers of quality filters have obtained AOA acceptance. When recommending AR filters to patients, it is effective to recommend they look for a product accepted by the AOA.

Privacy Filters

Some AR filters have the additional property that they do not transmit any light beyond a designed cut-off angle. When such a filter is placed over a computer display, the display can only be seen when viewed from a relatively normal angle to the surface (i.e., others cannot see the screen images when the user is seated before the display). This privacy feature is advantageous to many people such as human resource managers, executives, and air travelers.

Hoods or Baffles

A hood can be placed on the computer display to stop light from impinging on it. This is conceptually the same as placing a visor over the screen. By preventing light from hitting the screen, a hood likewise prevents reflections of that light. Typically, such hoods extend 4 or 5 in. from the display and protect the top and the sides of the display. A makeshift hood can be made by taping cardboard (or the file folder used for the test) to the computer display to serve as a light baffle. Hoods or baffles can be particularly useful where considerable light comes from an overhead light fixture or from a window to the side that can be effectively blocked in this manner. An advantage of hoods is that they do not decrease screen luminance as do AR filters. However, they often are not as effective because they block light only from limited directions.

Antiradiation and Antistatic Features

Many AR filters have a wire and grounding cord clip intended to be connected to grounded metal such as the frame of the central processing unit. This can help to reduce static buildup and also reduce the electrical field component (not the magnetic field component) of the extremely low frequency and very low frequency radiation coming from a CRT. It is highly unlikely that electromagnetic radiation is causing any problems for computer users so it is highly unlikely that providing such "protection" is of any real benefit; however, it is not harmful to use this feature, and it may provide some users with peace of mind. It must be emphasized, however, that AR filters are primarily used to provide visual benefits, not protection from electromagnetic radiation.

Final Note

Although AR coatings on spectacle lenses have visual advantages in general, they do not affect reflections in computer displays.

Summary—Diagnosis and Treatment of Reflection Problems

Diagnosis

Step 1—Specular reflections. Sit in the user's usual viewing position. Make sure your eyes are at the same height as the user's. Look for specular (mirror-like) reflections. Observation is easier with a dark background on the display. Note the source of the reflected light.

Step 2—Diffuse reflections. With detailed images on the computer display, shield the display from incident light with a baffle such as a file folder. If shielding improves the appearance or visibility of the images, then reflected light is problematic and should be addressed.

Treatment

SPECULAR REFLECTIONS

1. Remove the source of the reflections if possible. For example, use window blinds or turn off offending lamps. Other effects of these changes must be considered.
2. Tilt or rotate the display within reason to eliminate the specular reflection.
3. Change the workstation orientation in the workspace to eliminate the specular reflection.
4. Obtain an AOA-approved AR filter with a circular polarized feature.

DIFFUSE REFLECTIONS

1. Obtain an AOA-approved AR filter. Obtain a typical 30% transmittance filter if the display has adequate brightness; obtain a lighter filter if the display luminance range is limited.
2. Obtain a hood to place over the computer display. Use file folders as baffles to test effectiveness, even temporarily affixing with tape.
3. Reduce overall room illumination if it is too bright.
4. Consider replacing the computer display if it is too dim.

5. If the person is using bright characters on a dark background, switch to dark characters on a light background, if possible.
6. Obtain a privacy filter if indicated.

The role of the eye care practitioner (ECP) is to educate the patient about how reflections can affect vision when using a computer. Unless the ECP is conducting a workplace evaluation, the handout in Appendix 9-1 provides the computer user with a self-evaluation tool along with suggested management. Some ECPs offer the purchase of AR filters through their practice. Demonstrating the improvement on computer screens within the practice can convince the patient of the advantage of having one.

Chapter 10 reviews how the computer user can adjust the displays on their monitors to provide the greatest visual comfort.

References

Collins M, Davis B, Atchison D. VDT screen reflections and accommodation response. Ophthalmic Physiol Opt 1994;14(2):193–198.

Hladky A, Prochazka B. Using a screen filter positively influences the physical well-being of VDU operators. Centr Eur J Public Health 1998;6(3):249–259.

Scullica L, Rechichi C, De Moja CA. Protective filters in the prevention of asthenopia at a video display terminal. Percept Mot Skills 1995;80:299–303.

Wacker RT, Bailey IL, Tuan K. Visual performance on CRTs with anti-reflection coatings. Optom Vis Sci 1999;76(12s):268.

Appendix 9-1

Screen Reflections

Reflections in the screen decrease the visibility of text on the screen by decreasing contrast. You can determine if this is a problem by temporarily using light baffles, such as file folders, to shield the screen from offending light sources. If strong light is coming from overhead lights, 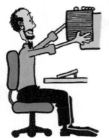 then use the baffle over the top of the computer display. If the light is coming from the side, such as from a window, place the baffle on the side of the screen.

If baffling the light results in a noticeable increase in contrast and clarity of the computer display, then the reflections are a problem and should be addressed.

One or more of the following can reduce your screen reflections:

1. An antireflection screen can be placed over the computer display. Look for an antireflection screen that has been approved by the American Optometric Association.
2. Eliminate the offending light sources. Windows and other bright lights behind you are the sources of the reflections.
3. Tilt or swivel thes computer display to eliminate the reflections.
4. Rotate your workstation to eliminate reflections.
5. Use dark characters on a light background. This polarity is less affected by reflections than are light characters on a dark background.
6. Place a hood over the computer display to shield it from offending sources.
7. Reduce the overall room lighting level.
8. If the file folder helped as a baffle, consider taping it in place.

More information is available at http://www.DoctorErgo.com.

10
Computer Displays

It is essential to examine the computer display itself—after all, this is the visual object that users are viewing when they are having visual difficulties. In some respects, the display on a computer screen is similar to a printed page. However, there are also several ways in which the computer display is different from paper displays, and some of these differences can contribute to difficulties in visual interaction with the task. The primary differences between computer displays and paper include differences in resolution, flicker, and contrast. Some of the differences can be easily observed by placing a printed paper on the screen, folded so that printed text can be seen immediately adjacent to screen text. This easily demonstrates that the image on the computer screen is not as legible as the image on the paper. The differences are even more pronounced when the comparison is performed with a magnifying lens.

One obvious method of improving the visual environment for computer workers is to improve the legibility of the display at which they are working. The role of the eye care practitioner (ECP) is to educate the computer user on the effect of poor computer display quality on their vision and give them guidance on how to maximize the display images.

Performance and Comfort of Computer Displays

Human performance and comfort are ultimately the most important measure of display quality. Early studies (Muter et al., 1982; Gould and Grischkowsky, 1984) showed that reading tasks were 20–30% slower on cathode ray tubes (CRTs) compared to printed paper. Increased screen resolution has generally been shown to improve reading speed, visual symptoms, or both. Jorna and Snyder (1991) measured reading speed differences that related to the image quality as measured by the area of the modulation transfer function. Harpster et al. (1989) showed better search performance with a higher resolution monitor. Sheedy (1992) showed that a group of 15 subjects read 17% more lines (P <.05) in a 30-minute reading session and reported significantly fewer symptoms on a monitor with 116.0 × 118.5 dots per inch (dpi) compared to a monitor with 73 × 80 dpi. It is clear that greater pixel densities result in better performance and comfort.

Human performance and comfort are related to the legibility, readability, or both of the display. Legibility relates to the ability to identify single characters and is similar to visual acuity. Readability is related to the ability to identify groups of words. Legibility and readability each involve sequentially higher levels of human interaction, interpretation, and judgment of the stimulus that is presented on the screen. Adequate resolution is a prerequisite for good legibility, and adequate legibility is a prerequisite for good readability. The legibility and readability of text can be affected by many variables such as font, type size, letter spacing, line spacing, stroke width, contrast, color, pixel density, gray scale, and monochrome versus color.

Sheedy and Bailey (1994) proposed and tested a legibility measurement method based on measurement of human visual acuity. The method is equivalent to using a visual acuity chart composed of characters or words of the particular design (e.g., the font style, stroke width, pixel density) for which the legibility is to be determined. However, an accurate visual acuity chart of the traditional design (i.e., progressively smaller lines of optotypes) cannot be presented on a computer display because the legibility of the letter decreases as it becomes smaller on the screen due to the inability of limited pixels to create a recognizable image. Therefore, in the proposed legibility method the characters or words are fixed in size, whereas the angular size is varied (to create different acuity rows) by having the subjects view the characters or words at a designed series of distances. The legibility method was used to measure the visual acuity of 10 subjects on each of six different displays. The same-sized characters were used on all six displays, and the mean acuity measurements on each display

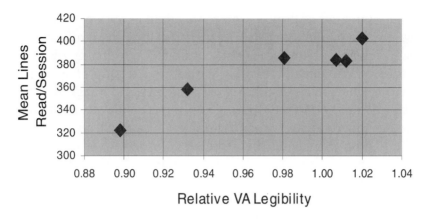

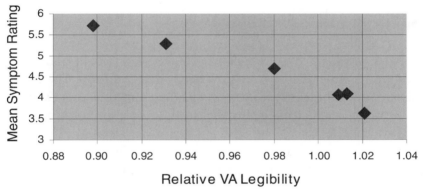

FIGURE 10-1. The relationship between relative screen legibility (as measured by the visual acuity [VA] method) and reading performance and comfort.

served as its relative legibility measure. In a separate study, reading performance and visual comfort of a group of subjects (21 subjects with a 20-minute reading trial on each monitor) were determined on those same six displays (Sheedy and McCarthy, 1994). The graphs in Figure 10-1 show the strong relationships between the relative legibility and the reading performance and symptom ratings; each data point is for one monitor. These results show that the legibility measurements made with a visual acuity method are positively related to reading speed and inversely related to symptoms.

The data in Figure 10-1 support the importance of viewing high-quality images for visual comfort and performance. The displays tested were representative of displays commonly used in the workplace, yet the image quality differences between them resulted in significant differences in reading performance and comfort. High-quality displays are therefore recommended. This also supports correction of small refractive errors, which likewise cause small decrements in image quality.

A simple method for comparing computer display legibility derives from the above. Place two monitors to be compared next to one another—each displaying the same text (same size, font, and other elements). Back away from the two monitors. The one with greater legibility and, hence, better performance and comfort enables text recognition from the greatest distance.

How Computer Displays Work

For many years, all computer displays have been CRTs (Figure 10-2), although flat panel displays are now becoming common. The CRT is a large vacuum tube with an internal electron gun that creates an electron beam. The electron beam strikes the phosphor coating on the inside of the CRT face. The electron beam is systematically scanned through the use of grids with electrical potentials across the inside surface of the CRT face. If the display is capable of 1,024 × 768 pixels,

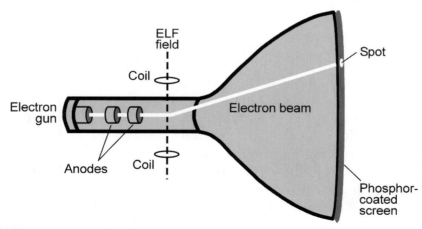

FIGURE 10-2. Schematic diagram of a cathode ray tube display. (ELF = extremely low frequency.)

then the electron gun is capable of being turned on or off up to 786,432 (832 × 624) times each time the screen is scanned. Each pixel represents a single picture element ("pixel" is a contraction for "picture element"). This is how the image is formed, by having the pixels either "on" or "off" each time the screen is "painted." If the screen is refreshed 85 times a second (refresh rate of 85 Hz), then the electron gun fires approximately 67 million times a second (786,432 × 85). This figure is called the *bandwidth* for the CRT; in this case the calculated bandwidth is 67 MHz.

A color CRT display has an additional level of complexity. To achieve color, the inside of the CRT face contains red, green, and blue phosphor dots. The phosphor dots are each activated by a separate electron beam. As the three electron beams scan across the display, a shadow mask is used to separate the three beams and allow each to stimulate their respective phosphor dots. The shadow mask is a curved metal plate with numerous small round holes through which the electron beams stimulate the appropriate phosphor dots.

In a color monitor, the spacing between the holes in the shadow mask is called the *dot pitch*. The size of the dot pitch is an important characteristic in describing the ability of a color monitor to display detail—smaller dot pitches are capable of displaying more detail. Also, because a portion of the electron beam is absorbed by the shadow mask instead of the phosphor, color displays often are not as capable of attaining the same luminance as monochrome monitors.

Flat Panel Displays

Flat panel displays are used in laptop computers and, as their cost decreases, they will likely supplant the CRT as the most common desktop display. Flat panel displays use liquid crystal display (LCD) technology, the same type of display used in wristwatches, pocket calculators, and similar products. Flat panel displays are much smaller in depth than CRTs because they do not have the bulky picture tube; the smaller footprint is a significant advantage for workspace arrangement. LCDs also provide a better visual image because they provide better contrast and do not flicker in the same manner as CRTs.

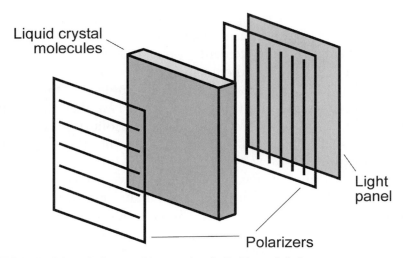

Liquid crystal molecules

Light panel

Polarizers

FIGURE 10-3. Schematic diagram of the operation of a liquid crystal display.

Whereas a CRT creates images by stimulating light transmittance from a phosphor coating, LCDs have a backlit panel of light that is selectively absorbed or blocked to create the images. The light does not continuously go through "on/off" cycles as with a CRT; hence, LCDs create significantly less flicker. An LCD can be simply characterized as having four layers: a back panel of white light, a polarized glass layer, an LC layer, and a second polarized glass layer (Figure 10-3). The polarization axes of the two glass layers are perpendicular; therefore, no light is transmitted unless the LC layer changes the polarization axis. The basic operation of an LCD hinges on the LC layer changing the polarization axis of light between the two glass layers. The change of polarization axis can be controlled locally so as to create a pixel of assigned brightness. Color can be created by having three controllable areas within each pixel, each with a small colored filter (red, green, blue) to create a spectral output.

LC molecules exist in a state that is between solid and liquid. The LC molecules are elongated or rod-like in shape. More specifically, the LCs used in displays are "nematic," meaning the molecules have an affinity to align with one another similar to a picket fence. Small microscopic grooves in the glass plates cause the LC molecules to align with the axis of the grooves. The axis of the grooves in each glass plate is the same as the polarization axis of the plate; therefore, the grooves of the two plates that bind the nematic LC molecules are perpendicular to one another. Because of the perpendicular grooves on opposite boundaries of the LC layer and the natural tendency of the nematic molecules to align with one another, the axes of the LC molecules gradually change their orientation, progressing from one glass plate to the other and resulting in a twisted "picket fence."

The twisted alignment of the molecules causes the polarization axis of transmitted light to likewise change; hence, the nonstimulated natural twisted alignment of the LC molecules changes the polarization axis of light by 90 degrees, thereby creating a white pixel. By applying an electrical potential to the pixel, the LC molecules straighten up and become aligned in one axis (in this configuration there is no change in the polarization axis), resulting in a black pixel. Gray pixels are created with partial voltage.

Resolution

Visual difficulties when viewing computer screens can be partly caused by the fact that computer screen resolution is poorer than most printed text. In optical terms, *resolution* refers to the ability to distinguish two visual objects from one another (Schapero et al., 1968; Millodot, 1986). The classic use of resolution is to distinguish two stars from one in a telescope. The smallest angle at which the two stars can be distinguished from one is a measure of the resolution of the telescope. For computer displays, the term *resolution* tends to be used more broadly. In common terms, the resolution of an image refers to the optical quality and density of the pixels on the screen and to the total number of pixels displayed on the screen.

The most commonly and easily obtained representation of the resolution of a computer monitor is the dot pitch, or the distance between pixel centers. For color monitors, this is the distance between same-color pixels. Smaller values are desirable; most monitors have a dot pitch of 0.28 mm or less. However, focus, convergence, and spot size also influence the monitor resolution. The ideal pixel would have a three-dimensional luminance profile similar to a pillbox or a cylin-

> **Box 10-1**
>
> Common dots per inch (dpi) values
>
> | Display source | Dpi |
> |---|---|
> | Computer display, dot pitch 0.25 mm | 100 |
> | Impact printer | 60–100 |
> | Laser printer | 300 |
> | Advanced laser printer | 600 |
> | Linotype printer | 1,200 |

der, in which all of the light was perfectly contained within the cylinder and there were complete drop-offs at the edges of the pixel. However, pixels do not have such a perfect luminance distribution and, instead, have sloping margins. One technical method of quantifying resolution is to assess the sharpness of the luminance edges of a pixel and express it with the modulation transfer function.

The pixel density on a display is directly related to the dot pitch—in other words, the dot pitch limits the pixel density and, hence, the fineness of detail. Box 10-1 compares pixel density on a high-quality monitor (dot pitch of 0.25 mm) to dot densities of commonly used printers. It can be seen that computer screen resolution is no better in the better impact printers. Impact printers are now seldom used and have been replaced by laser printers because of the noticeably better image quality. Computer screen resolution is fundamentally poorer than most printed text. This contributes to some of the visual difficulties when viewing computer displays.

Pixel Settings

The *video graphics card* is a circuit board installed within the computer that controls the number of pixels displayed on the screen. One of the earliest graphics adapters was the color graphics adapter, introduced by IBM in 1981, with 640 × 200 pixels. This was followed in

Box 10-2

Standard pixel settings

640 × 480	Video graphics array
800 × 600	Super video graphics array
1,024 × 768	Extended graphics array
1,280 × 1,024	Super extended graphics array
1,600 × 1,200	Ultra extended graphics array

1984 with the enhanced graphics adapter and with the video graphics array in 1987. The video graphics array is still commonly used today and has 640 × 480 pixels. The commonly available pixel settings are shown in Box 10-2.

Computer displays have one of the above standards as the maximum number of pixels that can be displayed. However, the display can be "set" to any of the lower standards by adjusting display settings through the control panel. It is instructional to adjust the pixel settings on your own computer. If, for example, you are currently operating at a setting of 800 × 600 and then adjust it to 1,280 × 1,024, the images on the screen become significantly smaller. This occurs because most images presented on a screen are composed of a given number of pixels. If the total number of pixels shown on the screen is increased, then the space occupied on the screen by a given number of pixels will necessarily decrease. Higher pixel settings allow more documents or windows to be seen simultaneously on the screen, but each is smaller. Users should select the setting that works best for them. Generally, settings nearer the middle of the setting options offer the best compromise between adequate size for reading and adequate space on the screen. For most users who must read text on the screen, it is important to set the pixels low enough that the image is adequately large for comfortable viewing. This can usually be set quite well by using subjective judgment but can be tested with the 3× rule described in Character Size and the 3× Rule and in Chapter 4.

Character Size and the 3× Rule

Text should be at least 3 times larger than the threshold size for recognizing it (basically the acuity threshold) for optimal performance and comfort. A technical method to test this criterion is to view the text on the screen from 3 times the usual viewing distance—it should still be recognizable from that distance.

The size of characters on the display is important for function and comfort. Size analysis can begin with the human visual acuity threshold. A 20/20 letter subtends 5 minutes of arc by definition. It is quite obvious, however, that the letter size needs to be larger than the threshold for identification. Research in the area of low vision indicates that performance improvements ensue up to the point that letter size is 2.5–3.0 times the threshold size. Applied to a person with 20/20 vision, this indicates a minimal letter size of 12.5–15.0 minutes of arc. However, further allowances need to be made for the image compromises inherent in computer displays and the fact that all users do not have 20/20 vision. Jaschinski-Kruza (1991) found that a group of subjects adjusted the screen viewing distance for 5-mm letters to a mean of 74 cm; this results in a viewing angle of 23 minutes of arc.

The 3× rule is relatively simple and can be applied to determine whether the character size is appropriate to the task and the person. The user should back away from his or her computer screen and determine the farthest distance at which he or she can just barely identify the text on the screen. This establishes the threshold size for that person. One-third of that distance represents the distance at which the text is three times the threshold size for that person; it also represents the maximum distance at which the person should be viewing the screen. For example, if the maximum distance at which the person can discern the text is 60 in., then he or she should be working no farther than 20 in. from his or her display. Although this viewing distance may be appropriate for the workstation, it is on the short side of normal. If it appears that the person is hunching too close to the computer, it may be because the text is not large enough or legible enough. The person may also be limited by his or her vision. Some complexities arise when using this test with users who are presbyopic, especially those who are older than 45 years. The 3× rule is only valid if the user is wearing appropriate refractive correction for the particular distance.

The 3× rule can be critical for senior patients. More and more retired persons are using e-mail to communicate with their children. Others enjoy games or surfing the Internet. Patients older than 65 years often have decreased visual acuity due to cataracts, macular degeneration, corneal disorders, or a combination of these. ECP counseling and proper prescribing must take into account the 3× rule, and ECPs must instruct patients on the proper image size and working distance. The working distance can influence the lens design and power prescribed as well as the viewing angle.

Screen Luminance

It is generally desirable to have a monitor with the capability of displaying high screen luminance. Although there are visual acuity gains and detection speed advantages by using higher luminance, the primary advantage of having the capability to adjust to higher luminance is to properly match the screen luminance to that of the visual surroundings. Also, if an antireflection filter is going to be used to enhance contrast, a higher maximum screen luminance can compensate for the luminance decrease caused by the filter. Please see Chapters 8 and 9 for more in-depth discussions of these issues.

Small improvements in vision have been shown with increased luminance. Ferree and Rand (1928) showed that the speed of detection increased for a series of sized targets as the illumination on them was increased. From these data and other studies (Lythgoe, 1932; König, 1962), it is clear that visibility increases greatly at the lower end of the luminance scale and that the visibility returns with increasing luminance are less at higher luminance ranges. Sheedy et al. (1984) quantified the effects of luminance changes on visual acuity and determined that over a range of 40–600 candle (cd)/m^2 every doubling of the luminance provides only one-fifth of a line improvement in visual acuity. This is equivalent to being able to identify one more letter on the smallest five-letter row at the subject's threshold size. For the range of luminance used on normal computer displays

($40–150$ cd/m^2), these small effects of increased luminance are not large.

The primary ergonomic issues concerning the display luminance are those of balancing the display luminance with other visual targets as discussed in Chapters 8 and 9. For these reasons, it is desirable for the monitor to have high-luminance capability.

Contrast

Of course, it is desirable to have high contrast on the display; this makes characters more legible. Contrast is typically limited by the darkness of "black" on the display. Better contrast is attained with darker blacks. Typically, the contrast is better with LCD displays than with CRTs. Because screen reflections play a large role in display contrast, this topic is discussed more fully in Chapter 9.

Contrast Polarity

Although the early CRT displays, as well as some current monitors or applications, use light characters on a dark background, it is usually better to use dark characters on a light background. A reason for the initial selection of light characters on a dark background was that the phosphors would "burn in" very easily. Another reason was that the 50-Hz flicker of early displays was very noticeable with black characters displayed on a green background instead of the opposite.

There are several advantages to using black on white, or the same polarity that is commonly found on paper tasks. It is not comfortable visually to view a dark object in the middle of a bright room. This is the situation with a dark background screen. With a white background screen, the brightness of the screen is a better match for the surrounding room (see Chapter 8). In fact, the best way to adjust the brightness of your screen is to adjust it so that it matches the background against which you are viewing the display. Also, dark background screens are prone to reflection problems. The reflections result in the entire background becoming brighter, therefore decreasing the contrast of the light characters on the dark background. With dark characters on a white background, the reflections do not reduce contrast or clarity of images nearly as much. With white background screens, it is possible to more comfortably operate in a normally lit office environment; with dark background screens, it is necessary to reduce the lighting in the office. Finally, studies have shown better work performance with light background displays (Bauer and Cavonius, 1980; Sheedy et al., 1990; Snyder et al., 1990).

There are a couple of situations in which the opposite polarity, or white on black, is advantageous. Some low vision users, especially those with media opacities, find it advantageous to reduce light scatter by using bright characters on a dark background. Low vision patients should be shown the effects of changing the contrast so that they can decide which contrast polarity works best for them. Another situation is one in which the user is not using the screen for continuous work but only needs to occasionally identify information such as on a stock ticker. In this case, visibility can be greater with the white-on-black configuration.

Gray Scale

As presented above, the pixel density on computer displays is sparser than that used for most high-quality printing such as laser printers. This results in displayed images with less-than-optimal resolution. In most applications, the pixels have a binary representation (i.e., each pixel is either black or white). One method of improving apparent image quality is through the use of gray scale imaging in which each pixel can have one of several gray scale values. Gray scale presentation of alphanumeric characters results in gray pixels forming many edge contours instead of jagged borders of black and white pixels. Naiman and Makous (1993) have demonstrated that thin, imperceptible gray strips can alter the perceived location of a black/white border, thus providing the theoretical basis for smoothing jagged edges and possible image improvement with gray scale. Sheedy and McCarthy (1994) determined that reading performance was 19% faster with a gray scale than with black and white pixels for a 100-dpi monitor and 7.3% faster with gray scale on a 120-dpi monitor; symptom ratings were also significantly lower with gray scale. It is clear that using a gray scale results in better performance and comfort.

Users seldom have the option of selecting gray scale. Most presentations of alphanumeric characters do not use a gray scale. Gray scale is most often used in the display of scanned images.

Screen Color

The color presented on a computer display is limited by the capability of the display and the graphics card. The number of colors that can be displayed depends on the number of bits used to create color. In the language of a computer, a *bit* is a single data element and can have a value of 0 or 1—that is, it is binary. If 4 bits of information are assigned to a single pixel, then 2^4, or 16, colors can be created. Many computers use 8 bits for color, resulting in 256 individual colors. More commonly, computers have 16-bit color (approximately 64,000 colors) or 24-bit color (three channels of 8 bits) resulting in 16.7 million colors. Most computers allow changing the color settings from the control panel. The highest setting gives the best color but usually compromises speed characteristics.

Most computer displays are color. However, if a display is dedicated to black and white tasks, then best image quality can be attained with a black and white display. This is because on most color displays three spots (red, green, blue) must be used to create each pixel, resulting in loss of image resolution.

One potential problem related to the color of the screen is that of afterimages. Some computer users have experienced the McCullough afterimage (McCullough, 1965). This afterimage results from the preferential adaptation of neural cells in the brain that are sensitive to visual borders. The McCullough afterimage was problematic on old screens with green characters on a black background; the green-on-black border detectors in the cortex (not the receptors in the retina) were excessively stimulated and therefore desensitized. Afterward, when looking at a white and black border, the white appears pink because the red-on-black border detectors are more sensitive than the green-on-black border detectors. This afterimage has been well studied and can last for a relatively long period—it can even last for days. Some people become quite concerned when this occurs.

Afterimages are seldom reported with current displays and only occur if a user views highly chromatic borders (characters). If a person has difficulty with the McCullough phenomenon, determine if he or she uses prominent colors on his or her screen. The afterimage problem can usually be resolved by changing the prominent colors the person uses. It can also be very helpful to turn down the brightness of the characters on the screen because dimmer characters are less effective at creating afterimages.

Flicker (Refresh) Rate

The image on a CRT computer screen is generated by an electron beam that stimulates a phosphor on the inside of the front surface of the tube. The electron beam scans the entire image line-by-line and thereby "refreshes" the screen numerous times a second (see How Computer Displays Work). As a result, each location on the screen is flickering and each pixel goes through numerous on/off cycles. The most common lowest refresh rate is 60 cycles per second (Hz), but higher refresh rates are usually attainable by current CRTs.

Flicker on LCDs is much less pronounced compared to CRTs. The light is provided by a steadily lighted back panel, the signal to a particular pixel only changes the transmission characteristics of a small filter. The signal is updated at approximately the same frequencies as on a CRT, but the only flicker that occurs is when the color or luminance characteristics of a particular pixel need to change. On an LCD, a steady-state stimulus on the display is not flickering, whereas it is continuously flickering on a CRT. Even when the stimulus must change on an LCD, the change does not entail a complete on/off as it does with a CRT—all that changes is the transmission characteristics of the small filter.

Human Flicker Perception

Human sensitivity to flicker is usually expressed as the critical flicker frequency (CFF). This is the flicker frequency rate beyond which we can no longer perceive the flicker. There is individual variation in

CFF, and the CFF also depends on various aspects of the visual stimulus. For most common viewing conditions, the CFF is in the range of 30–50 Hz. Because this is below the CRT refresh rate, we do not usually perceive the flicker. Flicker sensitivity can be decreased by selecting viewing conditions that lower the human CFF. Some of the pertinent visual conditions that apply to computer viewing follow (see Brown, 1965, for an in-depth review):

1. Screen brightness. A brighter stimulus results in a higher CFF. It is common for people to perceive the screen flicker on a computer screen (especially with a white background) if the brightness is adjusted high. By lowering the screen brightness and thereby lowering the CFF of the observer, sensitivity to flicker is decreased.

2. Screen location. The peripheral retina has a higher CFF and is therefore more sensitive to flicker than the central retina. Most of us can perceive the flicker of a white background CRT by looking to the side of it. The worker who continuously views a reference document placed to the side of the computer screen is more at risk for seeing flicker. Rearrangement of the workstation, brightness control, or both can help to alleviate this problem.

3. Screen contrast polarity. Larger flickering sources create a higher CFF than do smaller flickering sources. Therefore, human observers are much more susceptible to perceiving flicker with white background screens compared to black background screens; in this contrast polarity, the entire background is flickering instead of just the characters. Although this single factor favors the use of dark background screens, the balance of other factors strongly favors the use of white background screens.

Suprathreshold Flicker Effects

Although perceived flicker can be a problem for some CRT users, it is not a common complaint. The greatest potential problems of flicker are related to possible suprathreshold effects—that is, effects of flicker rates higher than our CFF and, hence, higher than our ability to perceive them.

At first it may seem unlikely that suprathreshold flicker could affect us, but this can quickly be dispelled by the fact that flicker-following responses can be recorded in the electroretinogram (ERG) at frequencies as high as 125–160 Hz (Brindley, 1964; Berman et al., 1991). Berman et al. (1991) measured the ERG on two subjects viewing a CRT with different refresh rates. Significant ERG responses, phase locked to refresh rate, were measured at 66 Hz for one subject and 76 Hz for the other. Synchronous ERG responses to fluorescent lights were measured as high as 145 Hz, and as high as 162 Hz for a physically modulated light from a slide projector. Eyesel and Burant (1984) showed that visual neurons in the optic tract and the lateral geniculate nucleus of the cat fired twice as strongly under fluorescent than under tungsten illumination and that the response to fluorescent lighting did not stop until they reached frequencies of 160 Hz. These results all demonstrate a retinal electrical (neural) response to flickering stimuli at rates considerably higher than we can perceive. Because there is a neural response to supra(perceptual)threshold flicker, it is at least plausible that it may contribute to symptoms.

Flicker-related changes in the visual system from working at a CRT have also been measured. Laubli et al. (1986) had a group of subjects work for 3 hours at simulated CRT displays with flicker rates of 30, 60, 90, 180, 0 Hz, and plain text. They measured the CFF before and after each session; there were clear decreases in the CFF after work with all conditions. However, the decreases with plain text, 0 Hz, and 180 Hz were nearly identical at an approximately 2-Hz decrease; the 60-Hz and 90-Hz displays created greater decreases (approximately 3 Hz); and the 30-Hz display created the largest decrease, approximately 4 Hz). Harwood and Foley (1987) had a group of subjects perform the same task on a CRT and on a back slide projection system (BPS). The only visual difference between the tasks was that the CRT was flickering and the BPS was not. The CFF of the subject population steadily decreased at 1, 2, and 3 hours of work on the computer screen whereas it did not change when working on the BPS. These studies indicate that something in the visual system fatigues as result of viewing suprathreshold flicker. This is further supported by Murata et al. (1991), who measured increased latencies in several peaks of the visual evoked potential after work at a CRT but not after work on hard copy.

Flickering stimuli also seem to affect our eye movements. Wilkins (1986) showed that saccadic eye movements were 11% larger when looking from one fixation point to another under 50-Hz flicker compared to 100-Hz flicker. Kennedy and Murray (1991) performed a similar study but with a task more similar to reading, and they also included a steady illumination condition. They concluded that flicker rates of 50 Hz and 100 Hz alter saccadic eye movements, reduce fixation accuracy, and increase corrective saccades. All of their data, however, are not completely consistent with those conclusions. Schweiwiller et al. (1988) studied the effects of 50-Hz, 80-Hz, and 100-Hz flicker on performance of a visual search task and were unable to measure a clear effect of flicker rate on task speed or error rate. However, Montegut et al. (1997) measured reading performance to be 3% faster with refresh rate of 500 Hz compared to 60 Hz. Tea et al. (1999) measured saccadic eye movement in 36 subjects who read text from a CRT display. Trial conditions included different colored overlays and refresh rates of 60 Hz and 70 Hz. Color overlays had no effect on saccadic movements, but there were significantly fewer saccadic regressions with 70-Hz flicker compared to 60 Hz. It appears that higher refresh rates enable more accurate eye movements and better performance.

It also appears that suprathreshold flicker is associated with increased symptoms. Wilkins et al. (1989) used a double masked design study to test frequency of headaches and eyestrain in normal fluorescent lighting (50-Hz lamps that produce 100-Hz flicker) and high-frequency ballast lighting (32 kHz) on a group of office workers. Even though there were no perceptible differences in the two lighting conditions, eyestrain and headaches occurred significantly less frequently with 32-kHz lighting than with 100-Hz lighting. It is not reasonable to expect that 32-kHz flicker is detected by the visual system. These results indicate that suprathreshold flicker (100 Hz) in fluorescent lamps contributes to eyestrain and headaches.

Clearly the human visual system is responsive to flickering stimuli at rates that are considerably higher than our ability to perceive them. Such suprathreshold responses have been electrically recorded from the retinas of humans and in the optic tract and lateral geniculate nucleus of the cat. Such suprathreshold flickering stimuli can cause measurable decreases in the CFF and can contribute to decreased performance and discomfort.

CRT displays commonly have refresh rates in the range of 60–90 Hz. The refresh rate of most CRT displays can be adjusted through software control panel settings. For optimal visual comfort it should be set to the highest refresh rate available; many people can feel immediate discomfort with a 60-Hz or even a 70-Hz setting. Decreasing the display brightness can also decrease discomfort associated with flicker. Flicker is not a problem with LCDs.

Epileptic Seizures

There have been some claims in the popular press that epileptic seizures may be induced by viewing a computer display (VDT News, 1993). Wilkins (1995) reports on a study of 170 photosensitive patients. Photosensitive responses in the electroencephalogram (EEG) were shown for frequencies ranging from approximately 5 Hz to 65 Hz. The peak was at 20 Hz; nearly all of the patients showed a convulsive response at this frequency. The percentage of the population dropped off both above and below this frequency; approximately half of the population showed a response at 10 Hz and at 50 Hz. Significant individual variation in frequency sensitivity was reported. He also reported that stimulation in the center of the visual field is more effective at inducing the effect than stimulation of peripheral vision.

Televisions have interlaced displays with refresh rates of 50 Hz in Europe and 60 Hz in North America; the interlace rates are 25 Hz and 30 Hz, respectively. These interlace rates are close to those that most frequently cause convulsive responses, and Wilkins suggests that they may be a causative factor. This seems very unlikely, however, because the amplitude of luminance flicker at the interlace rate is very low; the amplitude of luminance flicker is, by far, much greater at the fundamental refresh rate of the CRT. Wilkins also points out that most CRTs have higher refresh rates and usually are noninterlaced, therefore arguing that computer displays are less likely to induce seizures.

There are some reasons to suspect that the 8- to 12-Hz range may be responsible for inducing seizures. The 8- to 12-Hz range corresponds with the strong waveband that is recorded in the EEG with the eyes closed. This frequency range is also known to cause photic driving of the EEG. The center of this frequency range also has a period of 100 ms, which is a visual "constant" that appears in some fundamental visual processes such as the period of time over which brightness summation occurs.

Approximately 5% of people with epilepsy are photosensitive and many of them can self-induce a seizure by means such as waving fingers before their eyes or fluttering their eyelids (Binnie and Wilkins, 1997). Some seek these situations because they experience pleasurable sensations ranging from stress release to ecstasy to orgasm by doing so. This pleasure-seeking behavior can become compulsive and leads to self-induced epilepsy (Kasteleijn-Nolst Trenite, 1997). Some 150 self-inducing patients are described in the literature, and television displays are reported as being used by some of these self-inducing patients.

In a clinical report, Wilkins et al. (1999) reported success at reducing light sensitivity symptoms in some patients with photosensitive epilepsy by prescribing colored lenses. The hue and saturation of the color were selected using an "intuitive colorimeter." This instrument enables the patient to view a reading stimulus through a wide range of colored filters and to select the color that feels most comfortable. Twenty-three of 33 photosensitive epileptic patients reported beneficial effects during colorimetric testing and were prescribed colored lenses. Thirteen of the 17 patients available at 2-year follow-up reported benefits and were still wearing the lenses; 6 of the patients reported pronounced benefits such as reduced dizziness from fluorescent lighting and elimination of aura when viewing computer screens.

It appears unlikely that viewing a CRT display causes seizures, except perhaps in epileptic patients who self-induce their seizures. The refresh (flicker) rates of CRTs are higher than those known to cause seizures. The reported seizures seem to result from watching video games (VDT News, 1993). It is possible that some video games may have flashing lights and target movements that may, in some way, stimulate at the frequencies that may be causative of the seizures. If this is the case, it is not the fundamental flicker characteristics of the CRT but the flickering characteristics of the program that are implicated.

Laptop Displays

Laptop computers use flat panel displays; they have advantages of increased contrast and no flicker consistent with other flat panel displays. The largest concern about laptops is that the screen is attached to the keyboard, similar to the old video display terminals. This makes it impossible to simultaneously have both the screen and the keyboard at recommended ergonomic locations. For long-term use of a laptop at a desk, a hookup to a desktop monitor and external keyboard is recommended.

Virtual Displays and Head-Mounted Displays

Small high-resolution displays can be used close to the eye and can be viewed through optical systems that create a large viewable virtual image of the display. Such a virtual display can be presented to one eye in a hand-held device or two such displays can be mounted in a spectacle-type carrier, a form of head-mounted display (HMD). Such displays enable users to view common full-sized electronic files such as Web pages and word processing documents if the pixel count is adequate. Such displays are used for occupational and recreational (entertainment) purposes (Figure 10-4).

"Full immersion" HMDs completely block the wearer's view of the real environment, and the user is completely immersed in the virtual display. This is used for creation of "virtual reality," which is usually also accompanied by stimulation of hearing through earphones, and the screen images can be interactive with body movements through glove, head, or other motion sensors. "Partial immersion" HMDs allow the user to view a portion of the real environment and are more useful as informational displays for common work.

The viewing distance of the virtual image from the eye is set by the manufacturer, commonly at 1–2 m. Therefore, a person's distance correction is commonly required to clearly see the virtual image. If a person requires a distance correction, then he or she will likely require distance correction to clearly see the virtual image. Some HMDs can incorporate the user's optical correction into the device. For proper correction, the practitioner should know the distance of the virtual

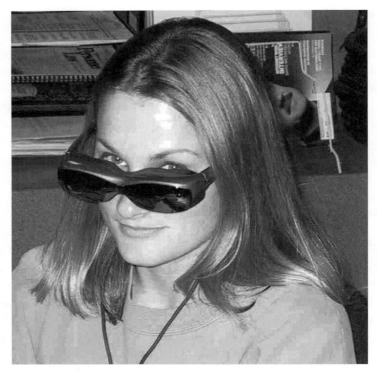

FIGURE 10-4. Example of binocular head-mounted displays, e-shades from InViso, Sunnyvale, CA.

image and provide a prescription for that distance. In most cases, it is the distance prescription; however, advanced presbyopic patients may require a small add.

Because HMDs can provide different images to each eye, it is possible to create a three-dimensional view of the world with disparate images presented to each eye. By converging their eyes, the user can have bifoveal fixation of objects at different distances. However, accommodation is not required in this virtual simulation of three-dimensional space because, even though the sensation of depth is created with disparity, the focal distance is singular for the entire scene. Users are required to converge without accommodating. This can be particularly difficult for patients with convergence insufficiency and for any patient for whom the negative relative accommodation finding (plus lenses to binocular blur) is less than approximately +2.00.

Another feature of HMDs is that the image moves with head movement, unlike the real world in which visual images move opposite to head movement. This causes discordance between the visual motion signals and the proprioceptive and vestibular motion signals. This has been shown to cause symptoms of motion sickness in several previous studies of HMDs (Mon-Williams et al., 1993; Regan and Price, 1994; Howarth and Costello, 1997; Morse and Jiang, 1999; Howarth and Finch, 1999; Hill and Howarth, 2000). In most of these studies, several subjects were unable to finish the trials due to symptoms. However, other studies (Rushton et al., 1994; Sheedy and Bergstrom, 2002) have shown that symptoms can be significantly reduced by using better-designed HMDs.

Patients who experience motion-related symptoms in traveling vehicles or on carnival rides are at greater risk for such symptoms while wearing HMDs. They are also more likely to experience such symptoms when using HMDs to create virtual reality environments or when viewing applications with considerable movement such as movies or games.

Summary

In summary, the role of the ECP is to educate the patient on how to achieve better visual comfort by using displays and display settings that provide the best-quality image. Appendix 10-1 provides a handout that may be given to the patient, enabling him or her to self-evaluate his or her monitor display and adjust the settings properly. Chapter 11 reviews the ergonomics of a workstation and gives guidelines on designing a workstation that results in maximum performance.

References

Bauer D, Cavonius CR. Improving the Legibility of Visual Display Units through Contrast Reversal. In E Grandjean, E Vigliani (eds), Ergonomic Aspects of Visual Display Terminals. London: Taylor and Francis, 1980;137–142.

Berman SM, Greenhouse DS, Bailey IL, et al. Human electroretinogram responses to video displays, fluorescent lighting, and other high frequency sources. Optom Vis Sci 1991;68(8):645–662.

Binnie CD, Wilkins AJ. Ecstatic seizures induced by television. J Neurol Neurosurg Psychiatry 1997;63:273.

Brindley GS. Beats produced by simultaneous stimulation of the human eye with intermittent light and intermittent or alternating electric current. J Physiol (Lond) 1964;164:157–167.

Brown JL. Flicker and Intermittent Stimulation. In CH Graham (ed). Vision and Visual Perception. New York: John Wiley & Sons, 1965;251–320.

Eyesel UT, Burant U. Fluorescent tube light evokes flicker responses in visual neurones. Vis Res 1984;24:943–948.

Ferree CE, Rand G. Intensity of light and speed of vision studied with special reference to industrial situations—Part II. Transactions Illuminating Engineering Society, May 1928;507–546.

Gould JD, Grischkowsky N. Doing the same work with hard copy and with cathode-ray tube computer terminals. Hum Factors 1984;26(3):323–337.

Harpster JL, Freivalds A, Shulamn GL, Leibowitz HW. Visual performance on CRT screens and hard copy displays. Hum Factors 1989;31(3):247–257.

Harwood K, Foley P. Temporal resolution: An insight into the video display terminal (VDT) "problem." Hum Factors 1987;29(4):447–452.

Hill KJ, Howarth PA. Habituation to the side effects of immersion in a virtual environment. Displays 2000;21:25–30.

Howarth PA, Costello PJ. The occurrence of virtual simulation sickness symptoms when an HMD is used as a personal viewing system. Displays 1997;18:107–116.

Howarth PA, Finch M. The nauseogenicity of two methods of navigating within a virtual environment. Appl Ergon 1999;30:39–45.

Jaschinski-Kruza W. Eyestrain in VDU users: viewing distance and the resting position of ocular muscles. Hum Factors 1991;33(1):69–83.

Jorna GC, Snyder HL. Image quality determines differences in reading performance and perceived image quality with CRT and hard-copy displays. Hum Factors 1991;33(4):459–469.

Kasteleijn-Nolst Trenite DGA. Dostoevsky's epilepsy induced by television. J Neurol Neurosurg Psychiatry 1997;63:273.

Kennedy A, Murray WS. The effects of flicker on eye movement control. Q J Exp Psychol 1991;43A(1):79–99.

König A. Die Abhangiskert der Sehscharfe von de Bekeuchtungsintensitat. In JPC Southall, H Helmholtz (eds), Treatise on Physiological Optics, vol 2. New York: Dover, 1962;369.

Laubli T, Gyr S, Nishiyama R, Grandjean E. Effects of refresh rates of a simulated CRT display with bright characters on a dark screen. Int J Ind Ergon 1986;1:9–20.

Lythgoe RJ. The measurement of visual acuity. Medical Research Council, Special Report Series No. 173. London: H.M. Stationary, 1932.

McCullough C. Color adaptation of edge detectors in the human visual system. Science 1965;149:1115.

Millodot M. Dictionary of Optometry. Boston: Butterworth–Heinemann, 1986.

Mon-Williams M, Wann JP, Rushton S. Binocular vision in a virtual world: visual deficits following the wearing of a head-mounted display. Ophthalmic Physiol Opt 1993;13(4):387–391.

Montegut MJ, Bridgeman B, Sykes J. High refresh rate and oculomotor adaptation facilitate reading from video displays. Spat Vis 1997;10(4):305–322.

Morse SE, Jiang BC. Oculomotor function after virtual reality use differentiates symptomatic from asymptomatic individuals. Optom Vis Sci 1999;76(9):637–642.

Murata K, Araki S, Kawakami N, et al. Central nervous system effects and visual fatigue in VDT workers. Int Arch Occup Environ Health 1991;63:109–113.

Muter P, Latremouille SA, Treurniet WC, Beam P. Extended reading of continuous text on television screens. Human Factors 1982;24:501–508.

Naiman AC, Makous W. Undetected gray strips displace perceived edges nonlinearly. J Opt Soc Am A 1993;10(5):794–803.

Regan EC, Price BA. The frequency of occurrence and severity of side effects of immersion virtual reality. Aviat Space Environ Med 1994;65(6):527–530.

Rushton S, Mon-Williams M, Wann J. Binocular vision in a bi-ocular world: new generation head-mounted displays avoid causing visual deficit. Displays 1994;15:255–260.

Schapero M, Cline D, Hofstetter HW. Dictionary of Visual Science. New York: Chilton, 1968.

Schweiwiller PM, Reading VM, Dumbreck AA, Abel E. The effects of display flicker rates on task performance. Proc Int Symp Teleoperation and Control, July 1988; 249–260.

Sheedy JE. Reading performance and visual comfort on a high resolution monitor compared to a VGA monitor. J Electronic Imaging 1992;1(4):405–410.

Sheedy JE, Bailey IL. Using visual acuity to measure display legibility. Society for Information Display International Symposium Digest of Technical Papers, Volume 25, Society for Information Display, Santa Ana, CA, 1994.

Sheedy JE, Bailey IL, Fong D, et al. Task performance and contrast polarity on hard copy and video displays. Proceedings of SPIE/SPSE symposium on electronic imaging science and technology. Society of Photo-Optical Instrumentation Engineers, Bellingham, Washington, February 1990.

Sheedy JE, Bailey IL, Raasch TW. Visual acuity and chart luminance. Am J Optom Physiol Opt 1984;61(9):595–600.

Sheedy J, Bergstrom N. Performance and comfort with near-eye displays. Optom Vis Sci 2002;79(5):306–312.

Sheedy JE, McCarthy M. Reading performance and visual comfort with scale to gray compared with black and white scanned print. Displays 1994;15(1):27–30.

Snyder HL, Decker JJ, Lloyd CJC, Dye C. Effect of image polarity on VDT task performance. Proceedings of Human Factors Society 34th Annual Meeting, Human Factors Society, Santa Monica, 1990;1447–1451.

Tea Y, Duong J, Ridder W. Effects of color filters and flicker rate on saccadic eye movements associated with visual display terminals. Optom Vis Sci 1999; 76(12s):132.

VDT News, March/April 1993.

Wilkins AJ. Intermittent illumination from visual display units and fluorescent lighting affects movements of the eyes across text. Hum Factors 1986;281:75–81.

Wilkins A. Visual Stress. New York: Oxford University Press, 1995.

Wilkins AJ, Baker A, Amin D, et al Treatment of photosensitive epilepsy using coloured glasses. Seizure 1999;8:444–449.

Wilkins AJ, Nimmo-Smith I, Slater AI, Bedocs L. Fluorescent lighting, headaches and eyestrain. Lighting Res Technol 1989;211:11–18.

Appendix 10-1

Computer Displays

The visual quality of the computer display can be very important for your visual performance and comfort. The following are some tips and suggestions about displays and how to use them to be as comfortable as possible:

1. Flat panel displays have visual advantages compared to cathode ray tube displays. They do not flicker and the contrast is typically higher.
2. Optimal contrast and visibility are attained with black characters on a white background. However, other combinations can be comfortable so long as the brightness contrast between the characters and the background is high. It is best to avoid dark backgrounds.
3. The size of the text should be three times the size of the smallest text you can read. You can test this by viewing the screen from three times your usual working distance—you should be able to read the text from this distance. If you cannot, then you should increase the size of the text or obtain an eye examination, or both.
4. The refresh rate (flicker) of most cathode ray tube displays can be adjusted (start/settings/control panel/display/settings). It is best to set the refresh rate as high as possible: 60 Hz is often too slow; 85 Hz or higher is recommended.
5. For color monitors, smaller dot pitches (less than 0.28 mm) are desirable.
6. Adjust the screen contrast so that the characters on the display are at their clearest.
7. The screen brightness should be adjusted to match the general background brightness of the room.
8. More information is available at http://www.DoctorErgo.com.

11
Optimum Workstation Arrangements

It is commonly recognized that "the eyes lead the body." Because working at the computer is a visually intensive task, our body will do what is necessary to get the eyes into a visually comfortable and efficient position, often at the expense of good posture and resulting in musculoskeletal ailments such as a sore neck and back. The various work location factors that influence comfort, visual efficiency, and body posture are discussed below.

Viewing Distance

The most common distance at which people view normal hand-held reading material is 40 cm (16 in.) from the eyes. This is the distance at which eye doctors routinely perform near visual testing and for which most bifocal or multifocal glasses are designed. Most commonly, the computer display is located at a farther distance from the eyes, 50–70 cm (20–28 in.). However, depending on the task and the individual, other working distances can also be comfortable.

In typical office situations, the effects of viewing distance cannot usually be isolated from other effects. In most situations, the text has a fixed size on the screen and the screen has a finite size to it. Increasing the viewing distance by moving the display farther from the eyes also results in smaller (visual angle) letters and a smaller (visual angle) screen. From a design point of view, it is possible to compensate for these problems by designing a display with a larger screen and larger letters that can be viewed at a farther distance. Much of the ensuing discussion on viewing distance considers it as a purely independent issue.

As discussed in previous sections, some of the difficulties associated with extended use of near vision are due to the extended use of ocular convergence (eye crossing) and accommodation (eye focus). Because a computer screen is usually farther from the eyes than typical reading, and the farther distance requires less convergence and accommodation, it is reasonable to expect that the greater computer display viewing distance would be more comfortable for vision. This concept is supported by a study (Jaschinski-Kruza, 1988) in which subjects performed work on a computer display at 50 cm and 100 cm; text size was compensated to be equal in angular size. Subjects reported less strain at and preferred the 100-cm viewing distance. In a subsequent study, Jaschinski-Kruza (1990) had 20 subjects perform a task that required frequent (every 2 seconds) fixations from the computer display to a reference document and back. He tested conditions in which the computer display and the reference document were both at 50 cm and in which the display was at 70 cm and the reference document at 50 cm. There was no difference in eyestrain between these two conditions. When the subjects were free to shift the screen to the most comfortable position (with the reference document fixed at 70 cm), they preferred screen distances of 50–81 cm with a mean of 65 cm. This argues for farther viewing distances for visual comfort, even if it necessitates frequent fixation changes between two viewing distances. Another study (Jaschinski et al., 1998) found that a group of subjects adjusted the screen viewing distance for 4.7-mm letters to a mean distance of 80 cm (range of 60–100 cm). It appears to be more visually comfortable to have longer viewing distances. This is reasonable because there is less demand on convergence and accommodation with farther viewing distances.

It has been proposed, and with some supporting evidence, that the greatest visual comfort is attained when working at the dark focus or dark vergence position of the eyes. However, Jaschinski-Kruza (1988, 1991) has shown greater comfort at 100 cm compared to 50 cm regardless of the dark resting positions. It appears that longer viewing distances are preferred regardless of the dark focus position—at least out to a 1-m distance.

Lie and Watten (1994) made various vision measures before and after 3 hours of work on two groups of subjects: one performing the work while viewing a computer screen and the other group performing the same work with audio input while viewing out a window. At the end of 3 hours' work, the computer-viewing subjects had significant increases in myopia and negative relative accommodation and significant decreases in positive convergence and positive relative accommodation. These findings indicate fatigue in the accommodative system expressed by less responsiveness and gravitation toward a fixed intermediate focus. The findings also indicate fatigue in ocular convergence ability. No significant changes were measured in the group viewing through a window. Viewing at a longer distance did not result in accommodative and convergence fatigue, indicating that longer viewing distances should be more comfortable.

Research supports that longer viewing distances are preferred.

Viewing Height

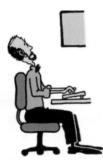

The height of the computer screen is a very important aspect of the workstation arrangement. The optimal height of the screen depends on several factors. Primarily, however, people adapt to the vertical location of their task by changing their gaze angle (the elevation of the eyes in the orbit), by changing the extension/flexion of the neck, or both. Therefore, these two postural elements are first discussed separately and then together.

Reference Planes

Before meaningfully engaging in a discussion of viewing height, it is necessary to establish reference points and planes for the head. The *line of sight* is easily established as being from the center of the entrance pupil of the eye to the fixation target. The fixation plane can be defined as containing the fixation point and the centers of the two pupils. The *horizontal visual line* is one that would pass through the center of the entrance pupil and a point on the horizon—or the same as the line of sight when looking at a point on the horizon.

The *Frankfurt plane* is often used to indicate the head attitude. This plane is defined as passing through the tragion (center of the ear hole) of each ear and the lowest point of the inferior ridge of each eye. Because it is highly unlikely that these four points are precisely located on the same plane, the definition is imprecise. However, for practical purposes, this defines a plane that can be determined. It is more accurate to speak of a *Frankfurt line*, in which case there is a right and a left Frankfurt line.

The Frankfurt plane requires palpation of the inferior orbit to locate a reference point. This can be awkward and difficult for both study and practical work, especially situations in which profile photographs are used to document head attitude. For this reason, it can be advantageous to use the *canthomeatal line*, which joins the external canthus of the eye with the external auditory meatus, or center of the external ear hole.

Jampel and Shi (1992) measured the Frankfurt line, canthomeatal line, and the horizontal plane by having a seated person place him- or herself in a position that felt neutral for eye and head positions. For a subject population of 28, the canthomeatal line was displaced upward by a mean of 14.95 (±4.02) degrees relative to the horizontal plane, and the Frankfurt line was displaced upward by a mean of 4.13 (±4.48) degrees relative to horizontal. These numbers (14.95 and 4.02) are important to convert and compare study data that report head attitude with the locations of these lines. Although the Frankfurt line is closer to horizontal than the canthomeatal line, the standard deviation of the canthomeatal line is lower, indicating that it is more accurately oriented with respect to horizontal than is the Frankfurt line. This fact, along with the relative ease of determining the canthomeatal line, argues for it being the preferred head attitude reference measure.

Ocular Gaze Angle

Hill and Kroemer (1986) had subjects adjust the vertical position of a reading task and determined that they set it an average of 28.6 degrees below the Frankfurt plane when the head was upright. This is converted to 24.1 degrees below the horizontal visual line. The preferred declination was greater when the subject was supine compared to seated upright, indicating a possible gravity effect on the preferred declination. They also found that the preferred declination relative to the Frankfurt plane was less (24.4 degrees) when the viewing distance was 100 cm than when it was 50 cm (32.8 degrees). These values are converted to 20.3 and 28.7 degrees, respectively, below the horizontal visual line. The finding of lower preferred declination with a greater viewing distance is consistent with other oculomotor findings, specifically the resting locations of vergence and accommodation (Heuer and Owens, 1989; Heuer et al., 1991).

Ripple (1952) determined that the amplitude of accommodation was greater with a downward viewing position compared to an upward viewing position. Changing from a straight-ahead position to 40 degrees of ocular depression, the eyes of 20 subjects became 0.99 diopters (D) more myopic, and the amplitude of accommodation increased by 0.7 D. The resulting near point of accommodation was 1.69 D greater in down gaze. These results were partially supported by Takeda et al. (1992), who objectively measured accommodation on three subjects and found a myopic shift of the far point but little or no change in the near point (thus, an actual decrease in the amplitude of accommodation) between the straight-ahead position and 16 degrees of depression. Atchison et al. (1994) measured the subjective far points and near points on 20 subjects aged 18–25 years; the results are presented in Table 11-1. They measured a closer near point and an increased amplitude of accommodation with ocular depression, but the magnitudes of the changes are considerably less than those measured by Ripple. They also made measurements on a group of 20 subjects aged 35–45 years and found little or no effect of ocular depression on the far and near points. The *straight-ahead gaze* was defined as the horizontal with the person in a head rest (i.e., with the chin and forehead in a vertical plane).

It appears there are some accommodative advantages to having ocular depression relative to straight ahead, and that these advantages are greater with 45 degrees of depression than with 20 degrees of depression. However, the gains in the near point of accommodation are quite small. Regardless, the accommodative advantages gained in

Table 11-1. Mean changes in far point, near point, and amplitude of accommodation with gaze angle

Gaze angle	Far point (D)	Near point (D)	Amplitude (D)
20 degrees up	0.17	−0.07	−0.23
Straight	—	—	—
20 degrees down	−0.05	0.15	0.21
45 degrees down	0.18	0.63	0.45

D = diopter.
Source: Reprinted with permission from DA Atchison, CA Claydon, SE Irwin. Amplitude of accommodation for different head positions and different directions of eye gaze. Optom Vis Sci 1994;71(5):339–345.

down gaze provide some rationale and support for the findings that people prefer lower gaze angles with closer viewing distances.

Sheedy et al. (1990) studied the editing performance of 25 subjects screened for good vision. The task was to count the number of occurrences of a specified letter in a nonsense paragraph as quickly and accurately as possible. Four trials were performed at each of six vertical gaze positions (30, 20, and 10 degrees down; 0, 10, and 20 degrees up) in randomized order. Performances were timed, and after each trial the subject was asked to rank the comfort of that vertical gaze position on a scale of one to seven, with seven being the most comfortable. Task presentations were photographs from a computer screen placed 50 cm from the eyes at a selected vertical position. The axis of rotation of the task was coincident with the center of rotation of the subject's eyes. Therefore, the subject's line of sight was perpendicular to the task at all viewing angles. A head and chin rest fixed the head location with the frontal protrusion of the chin and a point just above the brow line aligned in the vertical plane. The apparatus restrained the subject's head from tilting so that only eye movements were made.

Performance times and comfort ratings were normalized for each subject. The mean (standard error of mean bars) normalized values are presented in Figures 11-1 and 11-2.

The performance results show peak performance with 10 degrees of depression; comfort ratings were best with 10–20 degrees of depression. These findings were determined relative to the vertical

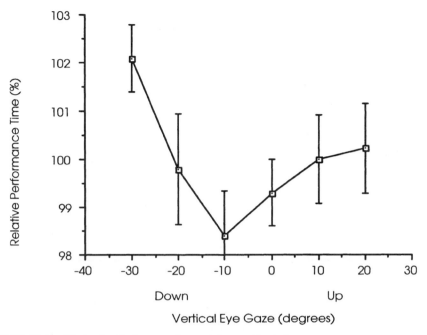

FIGURE 11-1. Effects of vertical gaze angle on a letter counting task.

plane of the chin and forehead; anatomic drawings indicate this plane is nearly perpendicular to the horizontal visual plane.

Some insights into ocular depression can be gained from the usual correction of presbyopia. The spectacles are fixed on the head, so only ocular movements are used to gaze through different locations of the lenses. Bifocal segments are usually located in spectacles so that the near viewing angle is 20–25 degrees below horizontal. This location has been empirically determined to be comfortable for most presbyopic individuals. However, if anything, it may be located toward the low end of acceptability because in the design and acceptance of bifocal lenses, consideration needs to be given to having a good field of distance vision, thereby encouraging the bifocal segment to be placed low in the lens.

In summary, all of these results certainly indicate better performance and comfort with ocular depression compared to elevation. For typical computer viewing distances, an ocular depression angle of 10–20 degrees relative to straight-ahead gaze (horizontal plane) seems

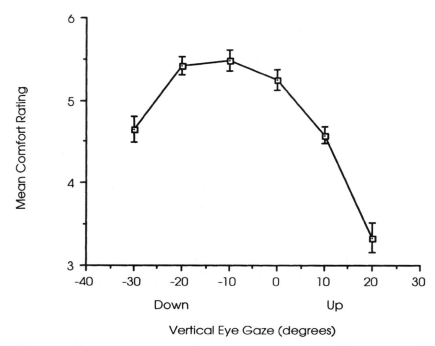

FIGURE 11-2. Effects of vertical gaze angle on subjective comfort rating.

indicated for optimal performance and comfort. However, there can be considerable differences between people regarding the preferred elevation and viewing distance of the display. It has been shown that users who can freely adjust the display location have a relatively small range of preferred settings. Locations outside of their preferred settings are less comfortable (Jaschinski et al., 1998).

Neck Extension and Flexion

Chaffin (1973) found that subjects could maintain flexion of the neck of 15 degrees for extended periods, but not 30 degrees. Kumar (1994) found that extension at the neck created discomfort. These results indicate that small amounts of neck flexion are preferred.

Total Display Height—Neck Flexion Plus Ocular Depression (Plus Torso Angle)

Small amounts of neck flexion and ocular depression are preferred; these would be additive in terms of their effects on the preferred height of the screen relative to the eyes. However, an additional element is the angle of the upper torso relative to gravity. For example, if the torso is angled backwards, such as when leaning back in a chair, then this would be subtractive to neck flexion and ocular depression in terms of its effect on screen height displacement (not the angle) relative to the eyes.

There is some reason to believe that the torso angle and the neck angle work to counteract one another. The head is relatively heavy and, to minimize the muscular effort to keep it upright, the body needs to keep it roughly balanced over the shoulders. For this to occur, the neck needs to flex forward as the torso tilts back. In a study of computer operators with adjustable workstations, Grandjean et al. (1984) found that 224 observers adjusted the workstation so that the screen center was an average of 9 degrees below the horizontal plane containing the eyes. This same group of subjects leaned backwards in their chairs by an average of 14 degrees, indicating that the sum of ocular depression and neck flexion was 23 degrees.

Consequences of Inappropriate Vertical Location

Adaptation to changes in display height can be accomplished by postural changes of the neck or torso or by an elevation of the eyes in the orbit. Sheedy and Parsons (1987) had 10 subjects wear 4 prism D of base down prism in front of both eyes that shifted the image of the world upward by 2.28 degrees. After wearing the prism for 2 weeks, the subjects had adjusted their measured head attitude upward by 1.74 degrees. This shows that most of the adaptation had occurred by postural changes rather than by ocular gaze angle change. The habitual position of the eyes in the orbit seems preferred over the habitual position of neck flexion. This lends further support to "the eyes lead the body." A similar situation occurs if the computer display is located too high or low.

Villanueva et al. (1996) measured postural adjustment of a group of subjects to a computer monitor located at a series of different heights. Over the 40-cm (approximately 39-degree) range of monitor height adjustment, neck angle changed by 25 degrees, eye gaze angle changed by 8 degrees, and thoracic angle by 5 degrees. Most of the adaptation to monitor height adjustment is accomplished at the neck.

If the computer display is located too high, most people tilt their head back so that they may maintain the usual and more comfortable downward viewing angle. This postural adjustment to a higher screen can cause neck and back aches. Because the preferred gaze angle is downward, a straight-ahead position of the display is considered too high. Other problems associated with a highly placed display are that the sources of discomfort glare (windows and fluorescent lights) are at a closer angle to the eyes and therefore are more bothersome. Another problem that occurs with a high display is that it results in a larger ocular aperture (greater exposed ocular surface), thereby increasing tear evaporation and exacerbating dry eye problems (Tsubota and Nakamori, 1993; Villanueva et al., 1996).

If the display is too low, it causes forward flexion of the torso and neck. This likewise causes neck and back aches. A low display also causes a person to provide some support of body weight with his or her arms on the work surface, potentially complicating wrist problems.

Screen Height Recommendations

It is clear that the screen should be located below the horizontal plane of the eyes. It is probably best that it be located so that it is 10–20 degrees below the eyes. This allows an appropriate amount of ocular depression. Neck flexion is compensated for by torso tilt, and this amount is consistent with preferences established by research findings. For practical workplace application, it is easiest to translate degrees into a linear measure of the height of the display relative to the height of the eyes. It is likely that the most commonly viewed part of the display is

Table 11-2. Height of display relative to eye height for 10 and 20 degrees of gaze angle

Angle (degrees)	Viewing distance in inches (cm)				
	20.0 (50)	24.0 (60)	28.0 (70)	32.0 (80)	36.0 (90)
10.0	3.5 (8.8)	4.2 (10.6)	4.9 (12.3)	5.6 (14.1)	6.3 (15.9)
20.0	7.3 (18.2)	8.7 (21.8)	10.2 (25.5)	11.6 (29.1)	13.1 (32.7)

the center; therefore, the optimal design rule should be applied to the location of the display center. Table 11-2 provides the height of the display center relative to the eyes at selected viewing distances to obtain 10 and 20 degrees of angle relative to horizontal. For example, at a viewing distance of 24 in., the display center should be 4.2–8.7 in. lower than the eyes to meet the 10- to 20-degree recommendation.

In some venues, it is recommended that the top of the display be at or slightly below eye level. Although not as precise, this recommendation usually results in a reasonable height adjustment.

Screen Tilt

There is little research support for a recommended screen tilt. When addressing screen tilt, it is most meaningful to represent it as relative to a perpendicular to the line of sight at screen center. A screen tilted away at the top provides an excyclorotation stimulus and tilted closer at the top, an incyclovergence stimulus. However, the literature does not clearly support whether adjustment to such stimuli is by vergence movement or by central psychosensory adjustment. Brand and Judd (1993) had subjects perform an editing task on a computer screen that was angled away at the top by 12 degrees from a perpendicular to the desk surface. Unfortunately, they did not specify the location of the eyes with respect to the screen, so it is not known what the angle of the screen was relative to the line of sight of the subjects. However, performance times and subjective preferences were better for the reference document being similarly angled (12 degrees) compared to conditions of 30- and 90-degree (flat on the table) tilt.

Hand-held reading material is typically oriented away at the top, providing at least some practical evidence that this may be a preferred tilt. In the absence of strong research support, it is reasonable to recommend that the screen be tilted to be either perpendicular to the line of sight or slightly away at the top. It must be remembered, however, that this recommendation is relative to a perpendicular to the line of sight at the display center. Because the recommended display location is 10–20 degrees lower than the eyes, the screen must be tilted away at the top by 10–20 degrees relative to a horizontal plane to be perpendicular to the line of sight. Hence, displays are typically tilted away at the top relative to horizontal and relative to a perpendicular to the workstation surface.

Reflections in the screen can be an over-riding determinant in recommending the best screen tilt for a given situation. In many environments, increasing the screen tilt results in increased specular and diffuse reflections. In these situations, adjusting the tilt to eliminate reflections, even to the exclusion of other considerations, results in the greatest gains in visual comfort.

Other Visual Arrangement

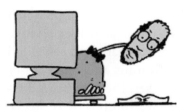 Whatever is viewed most often during daily work should be placed straight in front of the worker when seated at the desk. This applies to the computer, the reference documents, or both—whatever is viewed most frequently. Although this seems self-evident, many computer workers situate their work so that they are constantly looking off to one side.

The location of the reference material can also be important. Many computer workers place the computer display straight in front of them and then locate the reference documents on the table next to the screen. This is not very efficient. This requires large and frequent eye, head and upper torso movements to look back and forth from the reference documents to the screen. A good solution is to purchase a copyholder to locate the reference documents next to the computer display. An alternative design is to locate the reference document so that it is between the display and the keyboard.

Body Posture—How to Adjust a Computer Workstation

In-depth treatment of body posture is not covered. However, it is appropriate to mention currently accepted recommendations. Neck, back, shoulder, and wrist pain are common among computer workers. Sitting in one position for long periods of time can create such symptoms. Most studies suggest that frequent movement and change of posture is good. Although no single body position is good for long periods of time, it is useful to understand the seated posture, within normal office limitations, that is least stressful on the body. However, instead of structuring the following discussion around body parts, it is structured around office furniture and how it should be designed and adjusted; this allows the most useful way to apply the information.

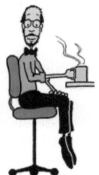

A computer workstation should be adjusted from the ground up (i.e., beginning with the chair height adjusted for the feet and legs). The following discussion is arranged in the same order recommended for adjusting a computer workstation.

- Chair. The primary chair features and optimal design/adjustment are as follows.
  - Legs/Rollers. Five legs are recommended, fewer legs are less stable and can tip over.
  - Height adjustment. Nearly all chairs have height adjustment. The height should be adjusted so that the feet are firmly on the floor, the thigh evenly supported on the seat pan, and the angle at the knee slightly greater than 90 degrees (i.e., the thigh should be oriented slightly downward from the hip to the knee). Shorter employees may require a footrest to allow higher chair adjustment.

- Back support. Back support is critical, especially lower back support. Some chairs have adjustable lower back support; it should be adjusted to the proper height for the person. Consider an ergonomic cushion for the lower back if unsupported.
- Back tilt. Some chairs have this adjustment. It should be adjusted so that the upper torso is bent slightly backwards (i.e., away from the computer display).
- Tilt tension. The chair should support the employee firmly in an upright position. If the chair tilts or rocks backward too easily, it can result in poor posture, especially neck strain. The tilt tension should be adjusted to maintain firm upright support.
- Armrests. Armrests are commonly absent or not used, often resulting in sore neck and shoulders because all of the weight of the arms is unsupported. This can also result in wrist problems because arm weight may also be supported with the wrists on the desktop. Armrests should have soft, rounded edges and should be adjustable in and out to accommodate girth and up and down. They should be adjusted so that the elbows, forearms, or both can be supported while keyboarding.
- Keyboard and wrists. The most comfortable position for the wrist is straight (i.e., no left or right bend) and extended 0–20 degrees upward. Adjust the keyboard height (if possible) so that the forearm is oriented slightly downward from elbow to wrist. A soft wrist rest in front of the keyboard can be helpful. Armrests should be adjusted to provide comfortable support for the elbows and forearms.

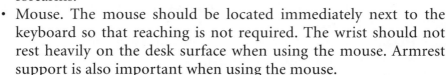

- Mouse. The mouse should be located immediately next to the keyboard so that reaching is not required. The wrist should not rest heavily on the desk surface when using the mouse. Armrest support is also important when using the mouse.
- Copyholder. A copyholder should be used to locate reference documents close to the computer display to avoid excessive head, neck, and even upper torso movement.

- Computer display. The height of the computer display should be adjusted so that the employee is gazing downward approximately 10–20 degrees. This can often be readily accomplished with old phone books or other props, although stackable spacers and mechanical support arms are also available.

Workstation Adjustment for Children

Scientific information is scarcely available on recommended posture for children. In the absence of such information, it is most reasonable to apply the same principles as for adults. The result is that computer workstations and furniture for children should be properly scaled to their body size.

Laptop Computers

Portability is the advantage of laptop computers. However, they are not optimally designed for long-term computer use, primarily because the keyboard and display are linked, thereby precluding both simultaneously being properly located for the body. For extended use of a laptop at a desk, an external keyboard or monitor is recommended.

Summary

Workstation arrangements can be critical to providing the proper visual angle and working distances to allow comfortable musculoskeletal postures. As an eye care practitioner, you are in a position to advise the computer user on proper viewing distance, viewing height, ocular gaze angle, neck extension and flexion, and screen tilt. Nearly all of the conditions that result in symptoms of discomfort also directly result in decreased task performance. An employee who is uncomfortable will not be as satisfied with his or her job and will become less productive. Visual discomfort problems associated with working at a computer can be solved by altering the environment to make it a more visually efficient and comfortable one.

Learning how to recommend the proper workstation arrangements enables you to serve as a consultant in evaluating workplaces. Appendix 11-1 contains a form that can be used with patients to communicate some of the most common and important recommendations in eye and ergonomic care. Chapter 12 builds on workstation arrangements to provide you with the skills necessary to become a workplace consultant.

Action Items

1. Train your staff on the importance of proper workstation arrangements for efficient vision and comfortable musculoskeletal posture.
2. Teach your staff to demonstrate the proper arrangements using an office workstation.
3. Develop a patient handout on how to properly adjust a computer workstation.

References

Atchison DA, Claydon CA, Irwin SE. Amplitude of accommodation for different head positions and different directions of eye gaze. Optom Vision Sci 1994;71(5):339–345.

Brand JL, Judd KW. Angle of hard copy and text-editing performance. Hum Factors 1993;35(1):57–69.

Chaffin DB. Localized muscle fatigue—definition and measurement. J Occup Med 1973;15:346–354.

Grandjean E, Hunting W, Nishiyama K. Preferred VDT workstation settings, body posture and physical impairments. Appl Ergon 1984;15(2):99–104.

Heuer H, Bruwer M, Romer T, et al. Preferred vertical gaze direction and observation distance. Ergonomics 1991;34(3):379–392.

Heuer H, Owens DA. Vertical gaze direction and the resting posture of the eyes. Perception 1989;18:363–377.

Hill SG, Kroemer KHE. Preferred declination of the line of sight. Hum Factors 1986;28(2):127–134.

Jampel RS, Shi DX. The primary position of the eyes, the resetting saccade, and the transverse visual head plane. Invest Ophthalmol Vis Sci 1992;33(8):2501–2510.

Jaschinski W, Heuer H, Kylian H. Preferred position of visual displays relative to the eyes: a field study of visual strain and individual differences. Ergonomics 1998; 41(7):1034–1049.

Jaschinski-Kruza W. Visual strain during VDU work: the effect of viewing distance and dark focus. Ergonomics 1988;31(10):1449–1465.

Jaschinski-Kruza W. On the preferred viewing distances to screen and document at VDU workplaces. Ergonomics 1990;33(8):1055–1063.

Jaschinski-Kruza W. Eyestrain in VDU users: viewing distance and the resting position of ocular muscles. Hum Factors 1991;33(1):69–83.

Kumar S. A computer desk for bifocal lens wearers, with special emphasis on selected telecommunication tasks. Ergonomics 1994;37:1669–1678.

Lie I, Watten RG. VDT work, oculomotor strain, and subjective complaints: and experimental and clinical study. Ergonomics 1994;37(8):1419–1433.

Ripple P. Variation of accommodation in vertical directions of gaze. Am J Ophthalmol 1952;35:1630–1634.

Sheedy JE, Kang JM, Ota WT. Vertical eye gaze position—effect on task performance and visual comfort. Unpublished, 1990.

Sheedy JE, Parsons SP. Vertical yoked prism—patient acceptance and postural adjustment. Ophthalmic Physiol Opt 1987;7:255–257.

Takeda T, Neveu C, Stark L. Accommodation on downward gaze. Optom Vis Sci 1992;69(7):556–561.

Tsubota K, Nakamori K. Dry eyes and video display terminals. Letter to editor. N Engl J Med 1993;328:524.

Villanueva M, Sotoyama M, Jonai H, et al. Adjustments of posture and viewing parameters of the eye to changes in the screen height of the visual display terminal. Ergonomics 1996;(39(7):933–945.

Appendix 11-1

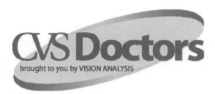

Improving the Ergonomics of Your Computer Workstation

To improve your comfort while working at your computer, we suggest that you particularly implement the changes that we have checked below:

Eye Treatment

_____ Use **artificial tears** as specified.

_____ Wear **glasses**, as specified, at the computer.

_____ Perform **vision training** as specified.

Computer Location

_____ **Lower** your computer screen so that the center is 4–9 in. below your eyes.

_____ **Raise** your computer screen so that the center is 4–9 in. below your eyes.

_____ Move your computer **closer** to you—best at 24–28 in. from your eyes.

_____ Move your computer **farther** from you—best at 24–28 in. from your eyes.

_____ Move your computer/reference documents to be **straight ahead** of you.

Lighting/Reflections

_____ Use an **antireflection filter** on your computer—preferably glass.

_____ Reduce bright **overhead lights** in your peripheral vision.

_____ Reduce the brightness of **windows** in your work area.

_____ Consider wearing a **visor**.

_____ Discontinue or modify the use of your **desk lamp**.

Workstation

_____ **Lower your chair** so that your feet are firmly on the ground.

_____ **Raise your chair** so that your entire thigh is firmly supported.

_____ Use **lower back** support.

_____ Use a **footrest**.

_____ Make room for your **legs** under your desk.

_____ Use a **document holder** to locate reference material close to the computer screen.

_____ Use a **wrist rest**/keep wrists straight.

_____ Properly use **armrests** on chair.

_____ Lower your **keyboard**.

_____ Locate **mouse** for easier access.

_____ Consider using a **hands-free** phone.

_____ Reduce **drafts or fumes** in your work environment.

12
The Eye Care Practitioner as a Consultant Providing Workplace Evaluations

An eye care professional who chooses to understand the ergonomic issues in the workplace can be very effective at providing on-site consultation for companies. Such consultation can improve employee visual comfort and performance. Opportunity for on-site consultation can develop as you provide specialized computer vision care to your patients and local companies become aware of your specialty. Or, a particular patient may be a human resources manager or safety officer and request that you become involved in helping to solve problems within the company. You can also promote such consulting services by establishing your expertise, promoting your expertise to your patients, writing articles for the local press, lecturing to interested groups within the community, or a combination of these activities.

Initial Meeting

Every work-site consultation is different, because every company, its employees, its environment, and the tasks performed are different. The first step in any evaluation is to meet with appropriate management at the company.

The primary purpose of the introductory meeting is to listen to the management's unique set of problems and what they want you to accomplish. You would not be there if there was not a problem to solve, and your principal activities need be directed at solving the problem. This initial meeting is your case history. There is a wide range of possible situations. Some examples follow:

- The company wants you to evaluate an employee who has filed a worker's compensation claim.
- A few selected employees are having problems.
- A new lighting installation is causing worker problems.
- The company wants advice on designing a new workplace.
- The company has just moved to new offices and wants to offer ergonomic and visual advice to those employees requesting it.
- The company wants to identify those computer workers who require special computer glasses.
- The company wants to implement pre-employment screening, etc.

At the initial meeting, you should endeavor to clearly understand their problem. You should also clearly tell the management what you believe you can accomplish and what you cannot. For example, you may be able to identify whether current lighting is good or bad and you can recommend how it can be made better, but you cannot specify the exact lighting system that they need. You should also ask about employee relations. Whenever you enter the workplace, you become an intermediary between employer and employee. You are likely to have been retained by the employer, so you should understand the employer's attitude toward the situation and the employees in general. Determine whether there are any legal or union issues involved. Ask whether you are free to talk with employees and whether there are any topics to avoid. In some situations, you will need to be escorted everywhere within the company; in other situations, the areas of concern will be shown to you and you will be free to navigate on your own. It is usually important to determine whether the company provides eye care benefits; if so, you should ask for plan details. Determine whether other experts have provided related consultation and ask to review a copy of their report.

Take reasonable notes at the initial meeting; this is the beginning of the consultant report that you will write. Exchange business cards with everyone at the meeting. It is useful to know the people and their titles. Depending on the situation, you may begin your evaluation immediately after the introductory meeting or schedule it for a later time.

It may be appropriate to survey employees to determine who is having problems. The questionnaire in Chapter 2, Figure 2-4, can be appropriate for this purpose. A tally of the results can indicate the extent of the problems and also indicate which employees require workplace visitation.

Before evaluating individual employees, determine the employer's policies and attitudes about paying for the following: eye examinations; computer glasses (i.e., glasses that are different from daily wear glasses); individual ergonomic items, such as antireflection (AR) filters, copy stands, wrist rests, and keyboard trays; and larger items, such as computer displays and chairs. You will want to use this information to guide your conversations with individual employees. You do not want to mention corrective items to employees that raise expectations beyond the employer's willingness to provide.

Before beginning your evaluations, you should have your equipment ready. The equipment listed in Box 12-1 can be useful. A camera (a digital camera is recommended) can be useful for including photos in your report. However, it is important to obtain approval from the

---

Box 12-1

Useful equipment for on-site evaluations
- Notebook
- Light-measuring equipment (luminance and illumination)
- Lens flippers to demonstrate adds and for accommodative facility testing
- Cover paddle
- Near visual acuity chart and near reading card
- Tape measure
- PD ruler
- Protractor, preferably clear plastic to see through
- Camera

employer and also from any individual employee before taking photographs. Some companies prohibit all photography on the premises.

General Office Evaluation

Before visiting individual employees, it is best to perform an overview of the office setting. This enables you to understand some of the primary factors and to have made observations and measurements before visiting individual employees. It is also likely that your report will be organized to include general office recommendations (e.g., lighting, window treatment, general statement about computer displays) as well as recommendations for individuals. Employees may be in individual walled offices, but it is more likely that most employees work in an open office with cubicles.

The following observations and measurements should be made in a larger office containing several computer-using employees. Appendix 12-1 is an example of a form for a general office evaluation. Employees can be very helpful in this process. Casually talk with them and ask necessary questions as you perform this analysis. Tell them you are making general measurements, but it is best not to become involved with the problems of individual employees at this stage.

- Note the light sources in the room. Tungsten, fluorescent, sunlight? If the room relies on sunlight, do people work at night? If so, you may need to revisit at night.
- Do the light sources (e.g., overhead fluorescent) create glare for a horizontal gaze angle in the room? Measure the luminance of the light source from an angle that is typical for a computer user in that office. Angles can be measured by sight with the protractor. Find the location of the light controls (switches) and determine what options and light combinations are available. If there are several options, try each, make luminance measurements, and form an initial opinion regarding the optimal settings.
- Is window light a problem? Measure the luminance of the window. Are window treatments available? Do employees use them? Are the window treatments (blinds, shades) effective? Measure the luminance when the window treatment is used. Pay attention to sun patterns;

open windows may be problematic only at certain times of the day. It may be necessary to visit at a different time of the day to evaluate.

- Walk through the office and measure prevailing illumination levels at desk level. Is it consistent throughout the office?
- Do the employees use localized lighting (e.g., desk lamps or under-shelf lights)? Does such lighting seem to be useful or harmful?
- Note the general posture of employees. Are the displays consistently too high, too low, too far away? This can be a good time to observe whether any employees engage in awkward head positioning, perhaps indicating inappropriate multifocal correction or a need for visual correction. Note the employees with such problems. Do the chairs seem to provide appropriate support? Are they generally adjusted properly? Are keyboards located at the right height? Do employees use reference documents? If so, are they located for easy viewing? Do employees engage in too much repetitive movement?
- Note the type of computer display(s) used. Liquid crystal display or cathode ray tube? Size? Measure the luminance range of the screen by adjusting screen brightness. Are screen reflections problematic? If so, can the source of the problem be corrected (e.g., open windows)? Do employees use AR screens? Are they effective? Measure screen luminance with an AR screen in place.

Indoor Air Quality

It is not uncommon to have poor air quality in a workplace (Backman and Haghighat, 1999). This is sometimes referred to as *sick building syndrome*. There is a significant relationship between poor indoor air quality and eye symptoms such as irritation, contact lens problems, and dry eye symptoms. Other common symptoms associated with poor air quality include headaches, respiratory symptoms, nasal congestion, dry or irritated throat, asthma, and drowsiness. Poor air quality should be considered in workplaces with high incidence of such symptoms.

Poor air quality can occur in any building, but is particularly common in newly occupied buildings, especially in which construction is still under way or in which new construction is occurring.

New carpeting, furniture, or draperies can also be sources of airborne irritants such as fire-retardant materials. Central ventilation disseminates irritants throughout the building. This also occurs if laboratories are not properly ventilated, causing poor air quality throughout the building.

Evaluation of Individual Employees

Assume the role of clinician when evaluating individual employees at their workstations. Your role is to determine the symptoms, screen the vision, determine whether the workstation ergonomics are adequate, and make recommendations. You should previously have obtained guidance from the employer regarding the items that will be provided for the employee. Individual employee evaluation at the workstation is similar to a clinical examination. A form for individual employee evaluation is at the end of this chapter (Appendix 12-2).

Typical objectives of the individual workstation assessment are to

1. Determine employee symptoms.
2. Determine whether eye care is indicated and indicate reason for referral.
3. Analyze the workstation ergonomics.
4. Recommend or implement, or both, workstation adjustments and changes to improve employee comfort.

If possible, try to first observe the employee at work without his or her knowledge. This can give a more accurate picture of habitual posture and work habits than asking the employee to assume his or her normal position when you visit. Note the employee's posture, especially head attitude and working distance, with special attention to awkward posture resulting from spectacle correction. Also note usage and placement of reference documents.

The employee should be seated as usual at his or her workstation. It is best for you to sit beside the employee. Evaluate each of the following areas as appropriate to the case:

- Case history. This step is significantly aided if the employee has filled out the symptom questionnaire. Ask about vision, eye, musculoskeletal, and glare-related symptoms (see Chapter 3). Also, determine the habitual corrective mode at the computer (no glasses, regular glasses, special computer glasses, contact lenses) and eye care history.
- Vision evaluation. The content of this part of the evaluation should be based on the symptoms, age of the employee, and your observations and measurements. The following areas should be considered:
  - Head and neck posture, screen height. This evaluation should be performed on all employees. Ask the employee to assume his or her normal position before the computer. If this is different than what you had previously observed, investigate the difference. Measure the distance from eyes to computer display. If it is unreasonable (usually between 50–70 cm or 20–28 in.), determine the reason, if any. If the employee wears multifocal lenses, determine whether the lenses are used appropriately or whether they are causing unacceptable posture. Measure the gaze angle (should be 10–20 degrees downward) to the computer display. This can be determined by measuring the vertical distance between the horizontal plane of the eyes and the center of the screen (should be 4–9 in. lower than the eyes for a viewing distance of 24 in.). The gaze angle can also be measured by viewing the employee from the side and using the protractor. Position the 0-degree axis of the protractor horizontal with the room and use a straight edge, such as the PD ruler, to point from eye to screen and note its angle relative to horizontal. Record whether the computer display is too high or low, and indicate whether multifocal correction seems inappropriate.
  - Visual acuity. Determine whether the person is adequately corrected for the computer display. Acuity can be measured with the near point card. Use lens flippers to test whether lenses improve display visibility; this can be particularly useful to test presbyopic needs.
  - Presbyopia. If the person is wearing a presbyopic correction, test whether it is appropriate for his or her work. Can the employee see clearly with a comfortable posture? Measure the range of clear vision through appropriate sections of the lenses. Use lens flippers

to test the effects of altering the add power. Lens flippers can be used to demonstrate benefits of an add to beginning presbyopes.

- Vision function. This area of evaluation is indicated in prepresbyopic individuals with asthenopic symptoms. Testing can include the following: cover test for near heterophoria, near point of convergence, amplitude of accommodation, accommodative facility test, or a combination of these.
- Dry eye. If patient symptoms and history indicate dry eye, make recommendations. These can include the following: lower the computer display if indicated, eliminate excessive airflow, improve humidity if indicated, teach the patient to blink when symptoms occur, use artificial tears, or obtain an eye examination.
- Lighting evaluation. For this evaluation, it is best to sit in the employee's chair to view the computer display as the employee does. Observe the display brightness compared to the general surrounding brightness—should the display brightness be adjusted? Determine whether glare sources are present (i.e., windows, overhead lights, desk lamps, 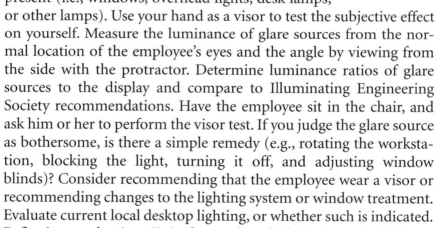 or other lamps). Use your hand as a visor to test the subjective effect on yourself. Measure the luminance of glare sources from the normal location of the employee's eyes and the angle by viewing from the side with the protractor. Determine luminance ratios of glare sources to the display and compare to Illuminating Engineering Society recommendations. Have the employee sit in the chair, and ask him or her to perform the visor test. If you judge the glare source as bothersome, is there a simple remedy (e.g., rotating the workstation, blocking the light, turning it off, and adjusting window blinds)? Consider recommending that the employee wear a visor or recommending changes to the lighting system or window treatment. Evaluate current local desktop lighting, or whether such is indicated.
- Reflections evaluation. Sit in the employee's chair. Use a file folder as a baffle to test whether blocking the impinging light improves display visibility. Determine whether the source of the reflections can be altered (e.g., turning off a light or using window blinds). Consider recommending an AR filter or hood for the display. Determine whether desktop surfaces are too bright. If so, measure the luminance and consider recommending a different surface or surface treatment.

- Computer display. You have already observed and measured the screen brightness and reflectance characteristics. Now judge the image size and quality. If the size is quite small, use the 3× rule test (see Chapter 10) to determine whether it is too small. If so, determine whether you can increase the size by changing the pixel setting or the screen magnification setting. Evaluate the color and contrast polarity of text; change if indicated and possible. If you can observe screen flicker (sometimes it appears to shimmer), evaluate the screen refresh rate setting. If there are significant and insurmountable shortcomings, consider recommending a new display.
- Body posture. Begin from the "ground up," as discussed in Chapter 11. Make and implement (where possible) recommendations for change as you evaluate. Adjust chair height for proper thigh support and angle at knee, and make sure the patient's feet are flat on the floor. Consider the need for a footrest for shorter employees. Adjust chair tension and back support. Evaluate keyboard position and height. Evaluate use of or need for arm rests. Adjust monitor height for proper visual angle. Evaluate need for copyholder or other work rearrangement.
- Furniture or workstation equipment. After evaluating the body posture and optimally adjusting the workstation furniture and equipment, evaluate whether the current equipment is appropriate. Significant shortcomings in chairs, keyboard height adjustment, arm rests, copyholders, and other items should be noted. Recommendations for new equipment or ergonomic accessories should be noted.

The most important part of the evaluation is the recommendations. These have accumulated as you have performed the above analysis. As in Appendix 12-2, first list workplace changes or counseling that you have already made. Then list any additional actions that are indicated, such as new equipment, ergonomic accessories, lighting changes, and window treatments. Use discretion in balancing the extent of the employee problem, the severity of the workstation shortcoming, the probable cost of the fix, and the employer's willingness to provide.

Determine whether the employee should be referred for eye examination. It is important to indicate the reason for the referral so that the examining doctor can have benefit of your evaluation; in this way, the patient is most likely to receive the appropriate care. Appendix 12-3 provides a separate form to be given to the referred employee.

Consultant Report

It is highly likely that your report will be shared with many others in the company—people whom you have not met and who have not been part of the discussions. It is therefore important that your report be both comprehensive and educational. You should define the entire process and include background and reasons for your recommendations.

As mentioned above, every consulting situation is unique. The approaches and forms in the appendices work in many situations but may need to be modified or may not work at all in others. Similarly, the organization of the report depends on the particular situation. The forms for general office and individual employee evaluation are not intended to be provided directly to the employer; they are intended for note taking and to serve as information sources for the report.

The following report organization follows from the approaches described earlier.

- Statement of the problem. This should be a succinct statement of the problem for which you were asked to consult. You may want to include a general paragraph about computer vision syndrome and its causes; a little education can be very useful.
- Procedures. Outline the steps and procedures you used to address the problem (e.g., met with specific company officers, distributed a symptom survey by e-mail, surveyed each office in general, met with individual employees who reported symptoms).
- Survey results. If you have surveyed symptoms of employees with a questionnaire, include it here to document the extent of the problem.
- General office issues. This section provides the foundation for most of the general recommendations you make to the employer. For each general area that you surveyed, include your overall analysis of the ergonomics. Include your lighting measurements, comparison to Illuminating Engineering Society recommendations, and your assessment of its adequacy. Also include your assessment of windows, work surfaces, quality of displays, general statement about furniture, and others.

- Employees evaluated. List the employees you evaluated along with a general statement about the types of problems they have had. It may be appropriate to tally the number of times each type of recommendation was made. Discuss if several employees are affected by office-wide issues such as open windows, poor lighting system, old displays, under-shelf lighting, poorly adjusted chairs, and high keyboards. Do not include analysis of or recommendations for specific employees; such information should be included in a separate report for privacy reasons.
- General recommendations. The above two sections provide the basis for the enumerated recommendations in this section. It may be appropriate to include discussion before the recommendations. For example, if you noted a lot of dry, irritated eyes and also that the air quality was low and that computer displays were generally too high, it would be appropriate to discuss this relationship before listing the recommendations. Include appropriate recommendations for lighting changes, furniture suggestions, policies on window blinds, eye care, ergonomic accessories, and others. Consider suggesting that you could give a lecture or seminar to employees about vision problems, proper workstation setup, and eye care. Be as specific as possible about your recommendations; they must be clear and actionable. As appropriate, suggest how you could assist in implementing your recommendations.

The analysis and recommendation for individual employees should be contained in a separate report. Information for each employee should be on a separate page. This enables the employer to communicate individually with each employee and also to freely distribute your report without revealing personal information.

Before finalizing your report, send a draft to your primary contact with the company. This gives the company an opportunity to suggest factual corrections and to identify any sensitive issues that you should discuss before finalizing the report.

Summary

Becoming a workplace consultant is a natural extension of your responsibilities as a computer vision specialist in your office. Following the suggestions in this chapter on evaluating the general office, evaluating the individual employees, and providing a report allows you to reduce office workers' stress in their work environment. You are able to improve the productivity of nearly every employee, resulting in an overall increased performance of the company. Many eye care practitioners have discovered on-site evaluations to be a fulfilling experience. Although much can be done to improve computer vision during an eye care practitioner examination, actually evaluating the workplace can provide you with the opportunity to deal with every factor influencing the comfort of computer use.

Establishing yourself as a computer vision specialist requires the proper marketing of your abilities. In addition to positioning your practice properly as discussed in Chapter 2, Chapter 14 provides guidance on developing a marketing plan. An eye care practitioner who wishes to provide evaluations at the workplace will require few changes to the marketing plan suggested by the chapter. On-site evaluations of workstations usually involve persons aged 18–65 years. Chapter 13 gives guidance on the examination and treatment of disorders affecting computer vision in children and senior citizens.

Action Items

1. Obtain and organize the equipment necessary for a workplace evaluation.
2. Review the General Office Evaluation form in Appendix 12-1, make any changes, and print on your letterhead.
3. Review the Employee Vision and Ergonomic Evaluation form in Appendix 12-2, make any changes, and print onto your letterhead.
4. Review the Eye Examination Referral form in Appendix 12-3 and make any desired changes.

Reference

Backman HA, Haghighat F. Indoor-air quality and ocular discomfort. J Am Optom Assoc 1999;70:309–316.

Appendix 12-1

General Office Evaluation

Office Location_____ Date_____ Time_____

General Room Lighting
Type
Source of glare?
Luminance

Windows
Location and treatment
Source of glare?
Sun patterns
Measurement

Illumination Levels
Locations
Conditions

Desk Lighting
Type
Glare source?
Needed?

Employee Posture
General
Specific employees
Furniture and equipment

Computer Displays
Type
Size
Reflections

Other

Appendix 12-2

Employee Vision and Ergonomic Evaluation

Employee name_____ Date of birth _____
Date_____

History
Symptoms
Vision correction
Eye care history

Vision
Head/neck posture
Acuity
Presbyopia
NPC, BV, accom.
Dry eye

Lighting
Glare sources
Luminance ratios
Desktop lighting

Reflections
Source
Treatment
Desk surface

Computer Display
Type
Size
Adjustment

Body Posture
Chair adjustment
Arms, keyboard, mouse
Display height

Furniture, Ergonomic Accessories
Chair
Keyboard
Other

Adjustments—Implemented

Additional Workplace Recommendations

Computer viewing distance is _____.
Eye examination indicated? Yes_____ No_____

If yes,
____General refractive ____Presbyopia—occupational correction
____Heterophoria ____Single vision for intermediate
____Convergence ____Intermediate/near bifocal
____Accommodation ____Occupational trifocal (large intermediate)
____Dry eye ____Occupational progressive addition lenses

Comments:

Appendix 12-3

Eye Examination Referral

Employee name_____ Date _____

This employee was screened at his or her computer workstation and has been referred for eye care for the following reason(s):

____General refractive ____Presbyopia—occupational correction
____Heterophoria   ____Single vision for intermediate
____Convergence   ____Intermediate/near bifocal
____Accommodation   ____Occupational trifocal (large intermediate)
____Dry eye   ____Occupational progressive addition lenses

Computer-viewing distance is _____.

_____
Referring doctor

13
Assisting Children and Low Vision Patients in the Use of Computers

Children

Computers are becoming a major part of the daily lives of children. A year 2000 national survey on home computer use in children showed the following (Lucile Packard Foundation, 2000):

- Ages 2–5 years: 27 minutes per day
- Ages 6–11 years: 49 minutes per day
- Ages 12–17 years: 63 minutes per day

As of 1999, the National Center for Education Statistics reported that 95% of schools and 63% of all classrooms have Internet access.

These numbers are certain to increase as computers become a more integral part of elementary education. However, even as school systems, government, and manufacturers rush to implement more computers in the schools, many others are expressing concerns about computers being harmful to children (Kelly et al., 2000; Alliance for Children, 2000); some are even calling for a ban on computers in the classroom until more is known. One group (Alliance for Children, 2000) lists the risks of computers to children as repetitive stress injuries, eyestrain, obesity, social isolation, and, for some, long-term damage to physical, emotional, or intellectual development. Obesity in children is linked to excessive time in front of a television screen— defined as 5 hours or more a day. The sedentary time spent in front of a computer screen could pose a similar risk. For most of these problems, hard evidence is not available. Very little research has been performed on children working at computers; however, given the importance of child health and learning, arguments for caution are weighty.

Some of the most significant concerns are not direct health problems, but the indirect harm caused by children viewing a computer for long periods of time instead of socializing and playing. A couple of catchy phrases include: "Two-dimension play is not as good as three-dimension play" and "For young children, seeing circles and squares is not as good as manipulating circles and squares" (Kelly et al., 2000).

Prima facie evidence supports concern for musculoskeletal problems. Although there are data and studies to support many of the ergonomic recommendations for adults, there are no studies specifically on the ergonomic requirements of children. In the absence of such studies, it is most reasonable to apply adult postural recommendations. This means that child computer workstations should be proportioned to children's body sizes; such furniture is not commonly available. Children have smaller bodies than adults, yet they often use a computer workstation designed for adults. In most cases, the display and keyboard are much too high, resulting in awkward posture. There is also no solid evidence to support musculoskeletal injuries in children resulting from computer work. However, it is possible that poor posture early in life can predispose to adult problems.

Vision Problems

Children can be subject to most of the same vision symptoms as adults. One survey found that 43% of children reported eye-related problems working at computers. Visual problems such as eye fatigue, eyestrain, burning eyes, tearing eyes, soreness, blurred vision, and headaches are all symptoms that are noted in adults and that can also occur in children. A special issue for children is that they may avoid performing the task if it is uncomfortable. This commonly occurs when children have difficulty with their eyes at near viewing distances. When they try reading, it is uncomfortable. Instead of becoming uncomfortable, they simply avoid reading, thereby harming their education. Of course, the symptoms are problematic, but learning avoidance because of the discomfort is potentially worse.

The development of myopia is a concern for some children. Clearly, the preponderance of myopia is genetically controlled. However, as reviewed in Chapter 4, there is reasonable research to support that some myopia development is related to performing extended near work with the eyes. No research has shown computer displays to create any more risk of developing myopia than other near tasks such as viewing paper.

Examination of Children

Symptoms in children should be assessed similarly to symptoms assessed in adults. Parents should be asked about school performance and whether the child avoids reading, other near tasks, or both.

Children who experience symptoms of discomfort or who present with a history of avoiding near work should have critical analysis of refraction, binocular vision, and accommodation. If the child is old enough to allow subjective responses, the testing, diagnosis, and management of these aspects of vision can be the same as presented in Chapters 4 and 5. In younger children, these functions can be assessed objectively with retinoscopy and cover test.

Children who begin progression into myopia should be closely observed. Binocular and accommodative function should also be assessed and treated when indicated. It is possible that esophoria, accommodative dysfunction, or both may be related to myopia development, and that treatment of these conditions may help retard the progression of myopia.

Virtual Environments

Head-mounted displays (HMDs) capable of creating virtual environments are now available and are likely to become used widely for games, entertainment, and work. HMDS are likely to become an attractive medium for children.

An issue of particular concern for most virtual environments is that the display moves with the head. As with adults, children could develop symptoms of motion sickness while wearing HMDs. Children who are prone to motion sickness during travel or on amusement rides may be at higher risk for developing such symptoms with HMDs.

As discussed in Chapter 10, virtual environments can create unusual accommodative-vergence stimuli. These areas of vision should be assessed in the presence of symptoms with HMDs.

Too much time spent in virtual environments may also affect development of spatial awareness. Basic spatial awareness skills are developed in infants and toddlers, but advanced spatial awareness skills, such as those required in sports, continue to develop into the teens. Concern has even been expressed about general computer usage and development of spatial awareness in children. This is highly related to the problem of spending too much time in front of a computer instead of playing outdoors. Again, hard evidence is lacking on this issue. It would be prudent to limit usage of HMDs in young children who are having difficulty with visual-spatial relationships. Such children show signs of poor sensory-body interaction with their environment and also often exhibit learning difficulties.

Recommendations

- Workstations for children should be properly proportioned to their body size.
- Children should have their eyes examined before beginning formal schooling.
- Any eye-related symptoms or avoidance of near tasks such as reading indicate a possible vision disorder and should be clinically investigated.
- Working, playing, or both at computers should be well balanced with a range of activities for full development. Parents should monitor computer usage to insure that the amount of time is not detracting from other important child-development activities.

Low Vision Patients

Blindness and visual impairment are increasing significantly as the population ages. According to the American Foundation for the

Blind, 10 million people in the United States are blind or visually impaired. The most common causes of visual impairment are age-related macular degeneration (45% of the low vision population), cataract, glaucoma, and diabetic retinopathy. For many low vision patients, it is extremely important to continue using computers for work, communication, and other daily living requirements. Rehabilitation for these patients can include optical, ergonomic, software, and hardware interventions. Some low vision patients have not habitually used computers, but the great adaptability of images on computer displays suits them well as part of the rehabilitation plan.

Recommendations

For low to moderate-low vision (20/60 or better), good function at a computer can often be obtained with typical presbyopic optical corrections by modest means. These involve increasing the screen image size by one of the following methods:

1. Go to the control panel/displays/settings and adjust the pixel settings. By adjusting the pixel setting to fewer pixels, the image on the screen becomes larger.
2. Many common programs, such as Microsoft Word and Excel, have a menu bar function that can change magnification of the document on the screen.
3. Increase the font size in text documents. This should probably be the last option because it changes the appearance of the printed document—unless, of course, the patient needs to print documents and requires magnification of the hard copy also.
4. Another means of obtaining magnification is to obtain a larger computer monitor.

Further magnification can be obtained by increasing the addition power in the spectacles. Because the computer screen is generally viewed with horizontal gaze, the higher addition power should be located in the lens center. An occupational progressive lens can work well because it also provides less add above and more below. A single vision prescription or a bifocal with the computer-viewing prescription in the top of the lens and reading prescription in the bottom of the lens can also work well. When a higher add (greater than approximately +1.50) is being used for viewing the computer screen, the patient should be counseled to move the computer display closer (i.e., it should be at the focal point of the add to avoid awkward posture). This can be difficult for adds beginning at approximately +3.00 diopters and ceases to be useful beyond approximately +5.00 diopters because it requires the patient to be too close to the screen.

If the above methods do not meet the needs of the patient, other options are available. Special screen magnification software can be useful. Such software has a full range of magnification settings, quick zoom features, special scrolling and mouse options, and contrast polarity and color settings. Such software can also "read" the text by converting it to sound. Several hardware and software devices are also available that use a camera and computer display to show magnified images of documents on a computer display. Some devices use a head-mounted camera and display to view a magnified image of distance vision for enhanced mobility. These devices will become more useful as camera and HMDs become smaller and the resolution becomes better.

Selected sources for computer-based low vision devices are listed in Box 13-1.

Action Items

1. Train staff to educate parents on the need for children to have a full eye examination before starting school.
2. Add questions to your patient history form for children to determine whether they avoid near work.
3. Counsel parents and children on the need to balance computer-game use with a range of activities for full development.
4. Learn how to advise low vision patients on how to adjust their display to allow comfortable viewing.
5. Train staff to demonstrate how to appropriately adjust the display in your office.
6. Prepare a handout on your letterhead informing patients of how to adjust their displays at home.

Box 13-1

Selected sources for computer-based low vision devices
http://www.visionadvantage.net
http://www.telesensory.com
http://www.freedomvision.net
http://www.optelec.com
http://www.magnicam.com
http://www.pulsedata.com
http://www.aisquared.com
http://www.clarityaf.com
http://www.enhancedvision.com
http://www.4access.com
http://www.jbliss.com
http://www.freedomscientific.com

References

Alliance for Children. Fool's gold: a critical look at computers in childhood. September 12, 2000. Available at: http://www.allianceforchildhood.net/projects/computers/computers_reports.htm. Accessed on May 15, 2002.

The David and Lucile Packard Foundation. Children and computer technology. Available at: http://www.futureofchildren.org/cct/index.htm.

Kelly K, Lord MC, Ma DL. False promise. Why computers fail as teachers—too much screen time can harm your child's development. U.S. News and World Report, September 25, 2000.

14
Marketing Yourself as a Computer Vision Specialist

Internal marketing always comes before external marketing, because if you market something you are not, your demise will occur faster than if you did not market at all. The patient entering your practice must experience what he or she expected from your external marketing. If the office does not appear computer-user friendly as communicated by your marketing, then you will lose credibility, and many potential patients will hear that you send misleading messages.

Chapter 2, Positioning Your Practice to Care for Computer-User Patients, discusses what is required to internally market your office correctly. Once you have carried out the suggestions outlined in that chapter, you are ready to announce to the world that you have something to offer computer users. To do this, you need a marketing plan. This chapter walks you through the steps required and gives examples you may wish to adapt to your particular situation.

Box 14-1 illustrates the steps required in developing a marketing plan (Moss and Shaw-McMinn, 2001). These steps will assist you in developing a marketing plan (Levinson, 1989), as in Box 14-2.

Step 1: Determine Marketing Goals and Objectives

Why do you wish to market yourself as a purveyor of computer vision services and products? Do you want more recognition? Income? Consulting opportunities outside the office? Often all three occur as a result of offering computer vision services and products in your practice. Complete the phrase "My marketing objectives are to" by choosing from the following:

Box 14-1

Steps in the marketing plan process

- *Determine marketing goals and objectives.* Use a practice mission statement for guidance.
- *Analyze the marketplace.* Assess your current situation and any barriers to achieve objectives. Use market research, data, and tools.
- *Identify marketing targets.* Analyze segmentation, targeting, and positioning of your present and potential patients.
- *Build long-term patient relationships.* Create a distinct eye care brand identity.
- *Manage the marketing mix.* Use the four Ps (price, product, place, and promotion) to gain competitive advantage. Use new technologies to promote your practice.
- *Understand product and service characteristics that patients value.*
- *Formulate a marketing plan and business strategy.*
- *Implement the marketing plan.* Develop benchmarks and controls.

---

1. Improve the compliance of my present patients with prescribed treatments relative to computer use.
2. Increase the number of computer-user patients by 104.
3. Educate the community so at least 50% of the people can explain how important good vision is to computer use.
4. Increase the number of computer-specific prescriptions by 200.
5. Serve as a paid computer vision consultant to five companies.
6. Increase the number of computer users completing a vision therapy program by 50.
7. Educate senior citizens on how they can best function on computers with less than 20/20 vision.
8. Cure 98% of my patients with computer vision–related symptoms.

Box 14-2

Marketing plan

Answer the following questions to give you a basic marketing plan.

1. The purpose of my marketing is to _____

2. I will achieve this purpose by focusing on the following benefits offered: _____

3. The target groups are _____

4. The marketing techniques I will use are _____

5. My image and brand identity will be _____

6. The budget I will allocate for this is _____

Many of these goals will be reached using internal marketing efforts and competent clinical care. Let us choose the second objective for our plan: *The goal of our marketing is to increase the number of computer-user patients by 104.*

Step 2: Analyze Your Marketplace

As you proceed with your marketing plan, you will learn that 90% of the plan comes from analyzing your marketplace. Statistics will indicate to you *where* you should market and *how* you should market. For example, if the Sally Mae Loan processing headquarters is in your community, every employee is a potential patient. You should focus your marketing efforts on that one company as opposed to 100 smaller companies. Complete a community analysis. Who is using computers? Who has the income to afford computer vision care? What companies offer vision plans that include computer vision care? How can you communicate with them? We know from Chapter 1 that there are 100 million computer-using workers in the United States and many more using computers at home. Are any of them near you?

Go to your Chamber of Commerce; local library; city, town, and county planning offices; and local phone books to get information to complete a community analysis. Use Appendix 14-1 to assist you in organizing the information. The information will allow you to recognize what patient populations you should target. You will discover where the computer-user workers are and which ones you wish to have as patients.

Consider referral sources. Who would be able to recognize computer vision problems and refer patients to you? Primary care physicians, orthopedic surgeons, pediatricians, nurses, school teachers, chiropractors, human resource managers, supervisors, government workers, older adult centers, computer stores, computer workers, office workers, information technology (IT) experts, legal secretaries, word processors, data entry clerks, accountants, and transcribers. Orthopedic surgeons, their nurses, and physical therapists commonly treat carpal tunnel syndrome experienced by many computer users. They can be an excellent referral source for you. Are there other eye care professionals who may refer individuals to you for computer vision care?

Analysis of the Woodcrest community shows that there are two main companies using computer workers: Pacific Telephone switchboard office and Amtrak reservation center. The elementary, junior high, and high schools have computers in every class. The only physician in the community is Peter Paul, M.D., and the only chiropractor is Melissa Springer, D.C. There are two real estate offices using computers. Potentially, many of the residents living in Woodcrest could be computer workers because most commute to work. There is a hospital 7 miles away and a water district office 6 miles away.

Step 3: Identify Marketing Opportunities

Look at your community analysis. Where are you more likely to get the 104 new computer-using patients you have targeted? What type of patient would you prefer to see? Do you want to see children who are using computers? Senior citizens who use computers? Computer-using workers? Is there a population you are not serving presently in your practice? Complete the patient profile exercise in Appendix 14-2 and compare it to your community demographics. There may be a segment of the community that you want to see that you have missed.

Woodcrest is seeing office workers from a hospital 7 miles away and a water district office 6 miles away but not from the telephone company or train reservation center. The physician sends patients for diabetes workups and eye disease, but not for computer vision evaluations. The chiropractor does not refer any patients.

Step 4: Build Long-Term Patient Relationships

The way to build loyalty is through practice brand. The eye care practitioner's practice brand comprises the sum of the patient's experience and features you and your staff provide to create a distinct, memorable identity of your practice in the patient's mind. Chapter 2 dealt with many of the factors that contribute to the practice brand, computer-user vision specialist. If you have not incorporated many of the suggestions, add them to your plan now. Whenever you make a practice decision, ask yourself, "Is this decision consistent with promoting the fact that this practice provides the best services and products available to computer-using patients?" Train your staff to use the same criteria when communicating with patients and potential patients.

Your brand as a computer-vision specialist is transmitted to patients through various media, including signs, print (brochures, letterhead, newsletters), visual symbols, staff uniforms, and mass media. An example of communicating this brand is the staff wearing a button saying, "Computer vision expert, inquire within" or "I care about computer users" printed over a red heart. A computer with glasses on may serve as a logo indicating your interests. You may wish to choose certain business hours to facilitate the appointment scheduling of your computer workers. Suppose the computer workers of a large company near you has a lunch hour from 12:00 PM to 1:00 PM. You may want to reserve this hour for examining their patients and take your lunch hour from 1:00 PM to 2:00 PM. If the company's typical work hours are 8:00 AM to 5:00 PM, you may wish to open at 7:00 AM or remain open until 7:00 PM.

You may wish to choose a theme to use that indicates your interest in computer vision. Woodcrest Vision Clinic: *computer vision services and products, your computer vision specialist, vision comfort for computer users, high tech for high-tech computer users.*

A patient will experience your practice brand in many different ways before, during, and after the actual encounter. All these influence points offer an opportunity to monitor and enhance the patient's perception about the brand image. Before any visit, word of mouth and referral sources that have been properly capitalized on can offer positive reinforcement. During the visit, the emphasis on catering to the computer user through staff communications, physical condition of the practice surroundings, examination procedures, and patient education material all have a direct bearing on the patient's perception of your practice brand. Finally, after the visit, you can solidify your brand image through follow-up communications, including phone calls, newsletters, surveys, e-mails, and recall notices.

At Woodcrest Vision Clinic, we emphasize computer vision brand by including computer vision services and products on all our marketing materials, offering computer vision information over our Web site, sending information to computer-using patients via e-mail, offering use of a computer with a digital subscriber line in our reception area, having staff scripts to use with computer-using patients on issues relevant to them, and offering computer magazines in the reception room, along with a computer game glassed-in reception area for children.

Step 5: Managing the Marketing Mix

At this point in the process, you must decide on four factors, referred to as the *four Ps*, of the marketing mix (Borden, 1965) by Professor Jerome McCarthy:

1. *Price*. Fees charged to patients and terms of sales
2. *Product*. Services and products the practice offers
3. *Place*. Physical distribution that makes products and services available to patients
4. *Promotion*. All communication activities the practice performs

Price

Fees you charge computer users should be on a level similar to other fees you charge until you become known as offering an expertise that is in great demand. After establishing yourself as a computer vision specialist with much to offer, you can increase your fees. The main determinate is whether your services and products are in great demand. Proper marketing provides this demand for computer vision services and products.

Product

What services and products do you wish to offer? Review the chapters in the book and decide what you are prepared to market. Will you offer a separate computer vision evaluation in addition to the basic eye examination? Will you offer a computer simulator examination? Variable focus lens designs? Monitor filters? Visual therapy? Daily wear contact lenses? Each of these requires office policies and staff training to be made properly available to your patients. PRIO now offers frames and lenses designed for computer users. Are you going to supply these? What about punctal plugs? Therapeutic pharmaceutical agents for conditions leading to dry eye? You must decide. Choose from Box 14-3 which services and products related to computer vision you wish to offer and set up policies and staff training to deal with them.

Box 14-3

Computer-related services and products

Computer vision–related services

Computer vision evaluations	Blink training	Fit 1-day contact lenses
Prescribe computer-specific lenses	Treat lid disease	Teach proper lighting
	Lid surgery	Teach to reduce reflections
	Treat ocular surface disease	Monitor display adjustments
Vision therapy	Treat ocular allergies	Workstation arrangements
Dry eye treatment	Fit low-water content lenses	Workplace consultations
Punctal plugs		
Punctal occlusion surgery		

Computer vision–related products

Progressive	Nonglare coat	Medicated drops
Variable focus	Scratch resistant	Oral medications
CRT trifocal	Tints	Antiglare screen
F/D or E/D	Aspheric	Document holders
Executive bifocal	Lubricating drops	Wrist pads
ST 35 or 45	Ointments	Back pads
Single vision	Lid scrubs	

CRT = cathode ray tube.

Place

The obvious answer to where to offer products and services is your office, but you may wish to offer computer vision evaluations at the patient's home or work. If you become a consultant conducting workplace evaluations for companies, your place just changed from that of your office. What do you decide?

Promotion

Much of Chapter 2 dealt with promotion. Research by the co-author has shown that once a practice is successful and booked in advance, no outside promotion is necessary. Word of mouth is sufficient to maintain and grow a practice. However, when offering new services such as computer vision, marketing to bring in new patients is necessary. Look at the marketing methods in Box 14-4 and choose which ones you are most comfortable with. Criteria for choosing them may include ease of implementation, cost, and expected return.

Step 6: Understand Product and Service Characteristics That Computer Users Value

This was addressed, in part, in Chapter 2. Here we will build on what is important to our computer-using patients. It is helpful to recall that patients do not buy our services but rather *solutions* to their problems. In your marketing, communicate that you have solutions available that will make their lives easier—at work, at play, and whenever they are using a computer.

How you and your staff feel will eventually be how your patients feel. Be sure to train staff properly and get their buy-in concerning the offering of computer vision services in your practice. Chapter 1 may be helpful in educating them to the importance of computer vision. Prescribing computer glasses or visual therapy for staff members may assist them in recognizing the worth of what you have to offer to computer users. Complete computer vision evaluations on your staff and prescribe appropriately. Experiencing the benefits of treatment such as computer-specific glasses allows them to give personal testimonials to patients.

Box 14-4

Marketing to bring in new patients

	Used successfully	Use needs improvement	Not using but want to use	Not appropriate
Direct mail	❏	❏	❏	❏
Newspaper inserts	❏	❏	❏	❏
Refrigerator magnets	❏	❏	❏	❏
Newspaper ads	❏	❏	❏	❏
Courses and lectures	❏	❏	❏	❏
School in-services	❏	❏	❏	❏
Seminars	❏	❏	❏	❏
Trunk shows	❏	❏	❏	❏
Medical practitioner referrals	❏	❏	❏	❏
Contests	❏	❏	❏	❏
Scholarships and awards	❏	❏	❏	❏
Community activities	❏	❏	❏	❏
Public relations	❏	❏	❏	❏
Clubs and associations	❏	❏	❏	❏
Outside signs	❏	❏	❏	❏
Reputation	❏	❏	❏	❏
Word of mouth	❏	❏	❏	❏
Tie-in with other professionals	❏	❏	❏	❏
Co-op funding	❏	❏	❏	❏
Radio ads/shows	❏	❏	❏	❏
Television ads/shows	❏	❏	❏	❏
Magazine ads/articles	❏	❏	❏	❏
Billboards	❏	❏	❏	❏

Always provide quality service. Research shows that above all, patients want confidence that they are getting what they need. Even if you make a mistake, correcting it quickly will be acceptable. Computer users want quality in a reasonable amount of time. Most work 8:00 AM to 5:00 PM at the very least. Their work often is stressful. They appreciate convenient hours and pleasant staff attending to their needs. "Service quality is the foundation for services marketing because the core product being marketed is performance. The performance is the product; the performance is what customers buy" (Berry, 1991).

The following practical tactics will assist you in providing the highest possible service quality:

1. Perform in-office patient surveys and focus groups to learn their perceptions.
2. Provide customer service training to members of the staff.
3. Anticipate patient expectations and then surpass them (e.g., a computer workstation with Internet access in the reception area).
4. Review and change any office systems that inconvenience patients. You may wish to be open during normal lunch hours.
5. Offer staff incentives to enhance service. Provide bonuses or "spiffs" to staff for each satisfied computer-user patient.
6. Focus on the functional quality of service that patients readily understand. They understand computers. Do a good job with your computers in the practice.

Review Chapter 2 and incorporate as many of those ideas as possible to make your practice computer-user friendly.

Step 7: Formulate a Marketing Plan

Based on the above process, your marketing plan will be the answer to the following questions:

Marketing Plan for Woodcrest Vision Center

1. The purpose of my marketing is *to increase the number of computer-user patients by 104 this year.*

2. I will achieve this purpose by focusing on the following benefits: *computer-user–friendly office design and policies; offering of all available computer vision testing methods; offer computer-specific products, including lenses, frames, and filters; offer computer vision syndrome treatments, such as punctal plugs, vision therapy, blink training, and workplace design recommendations; convenient hours during lunch and before and after 8:00 AM to 5:00 PM; and trained staff able to answer any questions on computer vision.*

3. The target groups are *Pacific Bell office, Amtrak reservation center, Parkview Hospital, Woodcrest water district, Peter Paul, M.D., office staff, Woodcrest Elementary School, Amelia Earhart Middle School, Martin Luther King High School, and children and adults who live in the community and use computers over 3 hours a day.*

4. The marketing tools I will use follow: *Design the office to be computer-user friendly, offer convenient office hours, give computer vision evaluations to my staff and Peter Paul, M.D., staff, and prescribe appropriately. Provide contests to the three schools on computer vision. Give in-service presentations to the teachers at the schools. Invite the human resource person from each of the targeted organizations in for a free computer vision evaluation. Offer to give a workplace evaluation for their private office space. Provide computer vision information displays at the libraries of the schools. Give seminars at the high school library on "Dangers of computer use," or "Vision and eye problems at computers"* (see Appendix 14-3). *Fliers to be used as newspaper inserts and distributed at the schools, Woodcrest community center, Peter Paul, M.D., office. Place newspaper announcement in local edition. Send letter to community homes introducing new services* (see Appendix 14-4 for examples).

5. My image and brand identity will be *computer-user–friendly office will offer all the services and products needed to competently solve the vision and musculoskeletal problems of computer users.*

6. The budget I will allocate for this is *10% of 104 × $300 (anticipated purchases per pt) = $3,120.*

It is often helpful to see the marketing plan laid out on a calendar. Box 14-5 is a sample marketing calendar for Woodcrest Vision Clinic.

Box 14-5

Marketing campaign calendar

Month	Activity	Cost
January	Take Peter Paul, M.D., to lunch; offer free computer vision evaluation to his staff.	_____
	Provide free computer vision evaluation to one of his staff members each month.	_____
	Invite human resource person from one of the companies for a free computer vision evaluation.	_____
	Computer vision library display.	_____
	Newspaper insert.	_____
February	Free computer vision evaluation to Peter Paul staff member.	_____
	Newspaper announcement of services and products for computer users.	_____
	Seminar at library: "Dangers of computer vision syndrome."	_____
	Electronic e-mail to computer-user patients.	_____
March	Free computer vision evaluation to Peter Paul staff member.	_____
	Middle school essay contest: "How do computers affect our eyes?"	_____
	Follow-up lunch with Peter Paul, M.D.	_____
	Staff training on computers and vision.	_____
April	Direct mailing to closest 1,500 homes to office concerning computer vision services and products.	_____
	Free computer vision screening.	_____
	Newspaper insert.	_____
May	Computer vision library display.	_____
	High school essay scholarship award: "How do computers effect our eyes?" Photo of winner with doctor in local paper.	_____

June	Seminar: "Dangers of computer vision syndrome." ____
	News release: "How computers affect our eyes." ____
	Send letters to local cable TV station, local radio station, clubs, and organizations offering to lecture on computer vision syndrome. ____
July	Mailing to human resource director at targeted companies. ____
	Electronic newsletter to computer-user patients. ____
	Frame and post latest testimonials from enthusiastic patients. ____
August	Staff training on computers and children, adults. ____
	Review office policies and procedures for handling computer-user patients. ____
	Update Web site and provide page on computer vision. ____
September	School in-service presentation. ____
	Back-to-school fliers. ____
	Take human resource person to lunch to discuss computer ergonomics. ____
October	Newspaper insert flyer on Computer Vision Help Web site. ____
	Elementary school poster contest: "How do computers affect the eyes?" Photo of winning poster, student, and doctor in local paper. ____
November	Trunk show: "New lens technology for computer users." ____
	Mailing to human resource director at targeted companies. ____
	Electronic newsletter to computer-user patients. ____
December	Refrigerator magnet with "Happy Holidays" greeting card to closest 1,500 homes to the office. ____

Summary

More and more of our patients are using computers daily. Soon the average patient we see will be a computer user. Providing computer vision services and products will allow the eye care practitioner to carry out his or her mission as a provider of eye care. Solving the problems of our computer-using patients will improve their lives and result in enthusiastic patients. Use the marketing information in Chapters 2 and 14 to communicate the benefits of what you have to offer to the general public. Learn from Chapters 3 through 12 and enjoy the satisfaction of one who has contributed to the betterment of others.

Action Items

1. Work through each part of the process in completing a marketing plan listed in Box 14-1.
2. Use the information gathered from Box 14-1 to complete your marketing plan as in Box 14-2.
3. Review the examples of marketing materials in Appendices 14-3 and 14-4 and adapt them to your situation.
4. Place your marketing plan on a marketing calendar.

References

Berry L, Parasuraman A. Marketing Services. New York: Free Press, 1991;5.

Borden N. The Concept of the Marketing Mix. In G Schwartz (ed), Science in Marketing. New York: John Wiley, 1965;386–397.

Levinson JC. Guerrilla Marketing Attack. Boston: Houghton Mifflin, 1989.

Moss G, Shaw-McMinn PG. Eyecare Business: Marketing and Strategy. Boston: Butterworth–Heinemann, 2001.

Appendix 14-1

Community Analysis

The purpose of this community assessment is to identify and organize certain facts about your practice community. From this community assessment, you will be able to get a realistic picture of the potential of your community for patients. The following sources may be used to get the information:

1. Local library
2. Chamber of Commerce
3. City, town, county planners (offices or committees)
4. Superintendent of schools
5. Social agencies
6. Local telephone books

Estimated population	_____	Number of families	_____
Percentage of age group mix		Number of households	_____
Infants (birth–4 yrs)	_____	Cost of housing (range)	
School-aged children	_____	Home ownership	_____
Young adults	_____	Rental	_____
Adults (26–40 yrs)	_____	% Of homeowners	_____
Middle aged (41–60 yrs)	_____	Type of transportation	_____
Older adults (61+ yrs)	_____	available	
			_____
Approximate annual income	_____		
% Of ethnic/racial mix		Number of office complexes	_____
_____	_____	Number of businesses	_____
_____	_____	Number of industries	_____
_____	_____	Types of industries	_____

Number of persons employed	_____	Number of senior citizen housing	_____
Number unemployed	_____	Number of nursing homes	_____
Major employers	_____	Hospitals, medical centers, clinics	_____

Types of work

Names of community leaders

Retail sales	_____	_____
Professional/technical	_____	_____
Computer	_____	_____
Heavy manufacturing	_____	_____
Light industrial	_____	_____
Clerical	_____	_____
Government	_____	Names of social leaders
Homemaking	_____	_____
Education	_____	_____
Self-employed	_____	_____
Executive/management	_____	_____
Others (specify)	_____	_____

Estimated school enrollments

Preschool	_____	_____
Elementary (grades K–6)	_____	Projected changes
Middle school (grades 7–9)	_____	Residential _____
High school (grades 10–12)	_____	Business _____
Trade school	_____	Industrial _____
College/university	_____	School _____

Appendix 14-2

Patient Profile

Patient's Name	Sex	Ages (yrs)					Occupations								Service rendered (by code number)*						Location (by quadrant or zip code)			
		1–17	18–24	25–54	55–65	65 +	Blue Collar	White Collar	Home-maker	Profes-sional	Retired	Stu-dent	Unem-ployed	1	2	3	4	5	6	1	2	3	4
Total																							

*Sample codes: 1 = diagnostic examination; 2 = contact lenses; 3 = low vision; 4 = vision therapy; 5 = glasses dispensed; 6 = computer-user examination.

Appendix 14-3

Vision and Eye Problems at Computers

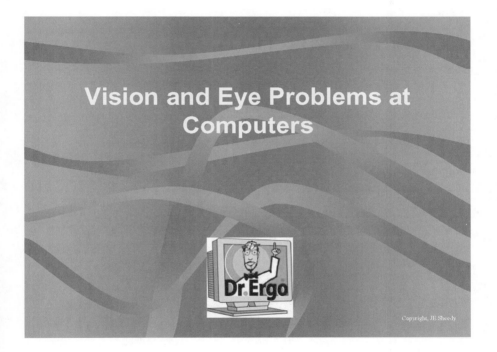

Computer Vision Syndrome

"The complex of eye and vision problems related to near work which are experienced during or related to computer use"

American Optometric Association

Copyright, JE Sheedy

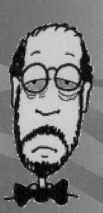

Eye problems are primarily symptomatic

Copyright, JE Sheedy

The most common symptoms

- eye strain
- headaches
- blurred vision
- dry, irritated eyes
- neck ache
- back ache

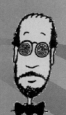

Reasons for Symptoms

- eye disorder
- workplace disorder
- combination

CVS - Causative Vision and Eye Conditions

- Refractive errors
- Accommodative disorders
- Binocular vision disorders
- Dry eyes
- Presbyopia and its correction

Copyright, JE Sheedy

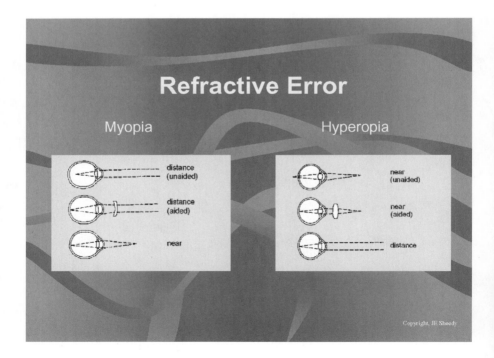

Refractive Error

Myopia   Hyperopia

Copyright, JE Sheedy

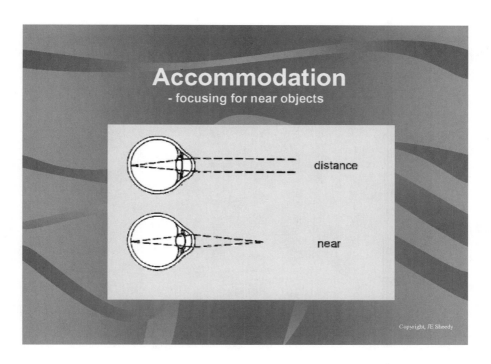

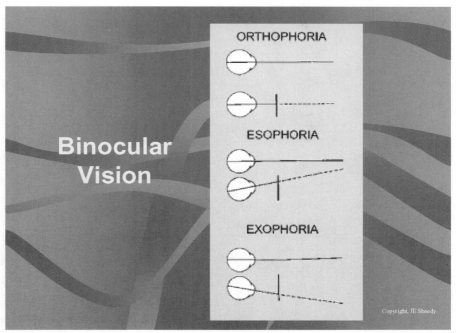

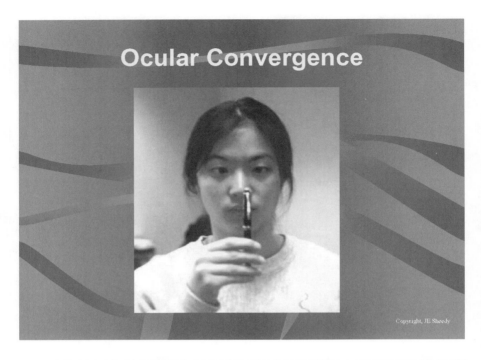

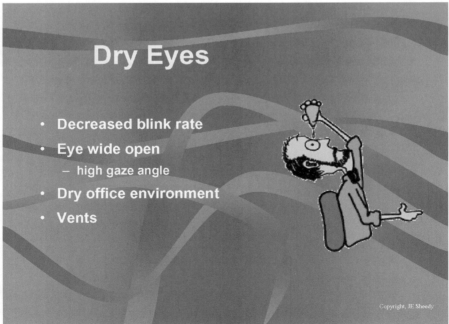

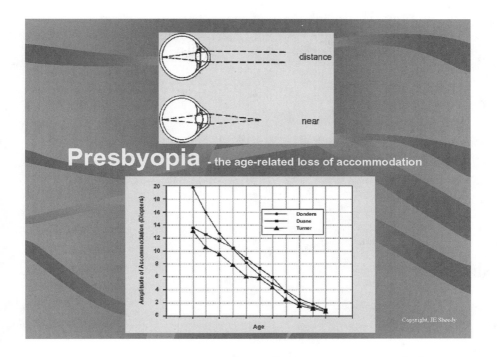

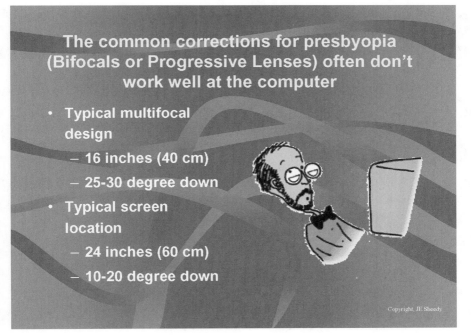

- when your "normal" glasses don't work
well at the computer

- • Special occupational lenses
  - – emphasis on intermediate power

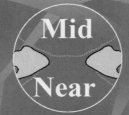

Lens Options for the Computer

- • **Tinted Lenses at the Computer**
  - – Most are cosmetic
  - – Pink may provide some comfort in fluorescent lighting
- • **UV protection for computer users**
  - – no need
  - – no UV hazard at the computer
- • **Anti-reflection coatings**
  - – Improve vision generally
  - – Helpful for performing critical tasks

Computer glasses - requirements

American Optometric Association

- **Would not require the glasses for a less demanding visual job**
  - hyperopia
  - astigmatism
  - heterophoria
  - accommodative dysfunction
- **Glasses at computer are different in power or design than those for most daily visual needs**
  - presbyopia

Copyright, JE Sheedy

The computer work environment

Copyright, JE Sheedy

Fundamental lighting principle

Good quality lighting entails having relatively equal luminances (brightnesses) in the field of view

Copyright, JE Sheedy

Lighting

- **Bright lights cause discomfort**

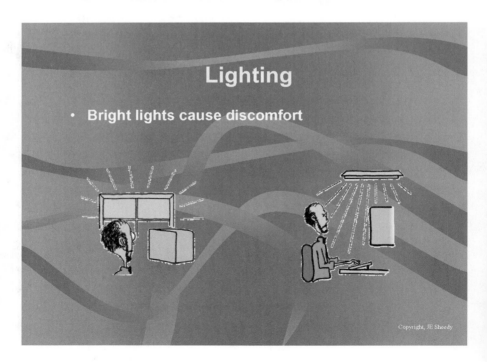

Copyright, JE Sheedy

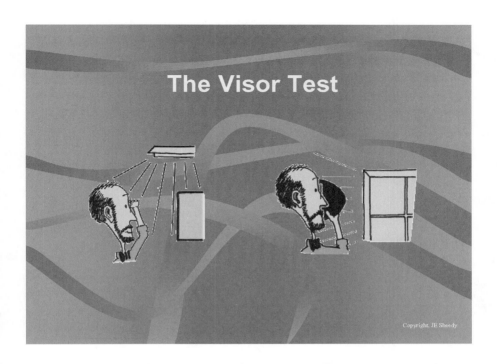

The Visor Test

Copyright, JE Sheedy

Improving lighting

- turn off some lights
- blinds/drapes
- remove white surfaces
- fix auxiliary lighting
- partitions
- rotate work station
- down lighting
- indirect lighting
- wear a visor

Copyright, JE Sheedy

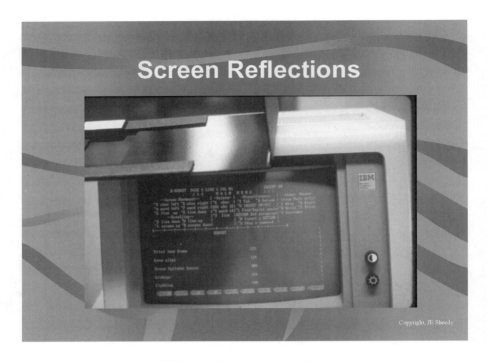

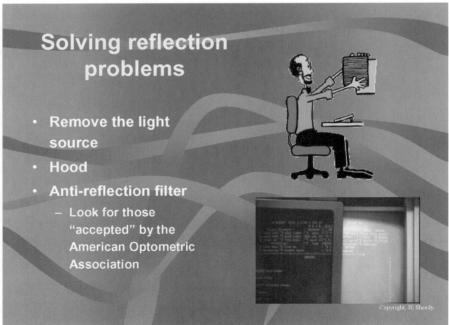

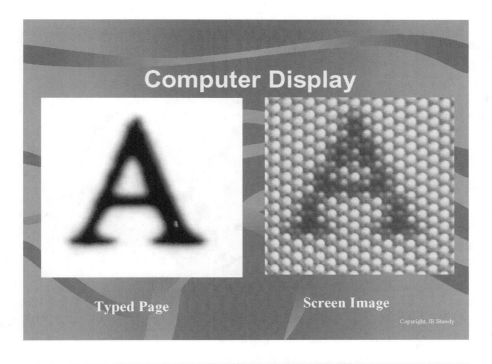

Computer Display

Typed Page

Screen Image

Copyright, JE Sheedy

Important Display Characteristics

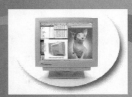

- Larger screens are generally better
  - can display higher pixel formats with an adequate size
- LCD displays are generally better
  - no flicker
  - good clarity
- Adjust brightness to match surrounding room in field of view

Copyright, JE Sheedy

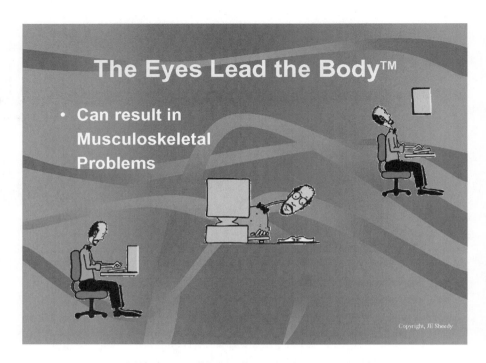

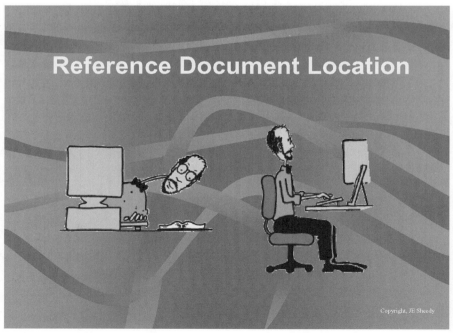

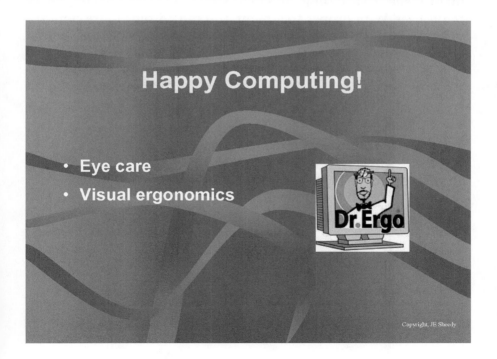

Appendix 14-4

Examples of Marketing Materials

COMPUTER VISION HELP WEB PAGE

An update on the latest advances in computer vision syndrome diagnosis and treatment is now available by checking the Computer Vision Help Web Page at http://www.Massengillvisioncenter.com.

You will receive information on the indications, benefits, alternatives, and risks of treatments for computer vision syndrome, as well as help on reducing the costs and stress of necessary procedures.

The goal of Computer Vision Help Web Page is to dispel some of the many misunderstandings and myths about the effect of computers on the eyes. With proper treatment, you can become more comfortable, experience less stress, and increase performance when working on a computer.

Computer Vision Help Web Page is presented as a public service by the Massengill Vision Center.

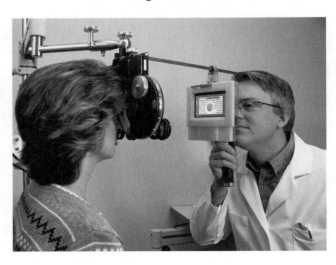

MODERN COMPUTER VISION

Computer vision is one of the most dynamic fields in all of eye care, with frequent new advances. Current techniques feature computer simulators and high technology, as well as innovations in lens designs.

Our services now include computer vision workplace evaluations in your place of employment or home workstation.

If you have a significant visual handicap because of computer vision syndrome, many options are available to improve your comfort, depending on what is in your best interest.

J. F. MASSENGILL VISION CENTER
Pacific Coast Medical Clinic
27830 Bradley Road
San Diego, California 92128
(760) 695-2020
http://www.Massengillvisioncenter.com

Certified by Computer Vision Syndrome doctors: Graduate, University of California at Berkeley Optometry School; member, Computer Vision Syndrome Doctors, San Diego Optometric Society, San Diego Eye Bank, San Diego Prevent Blindness Association Chapter

FREE COMPUTER VISION SCREENING

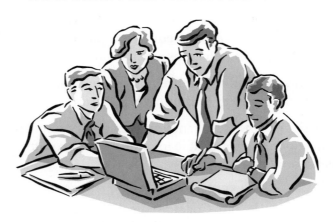

Computer vision syndrome is a common cause of eye discomfort and reduced vision. If you have significant problems related to computer use, a free screening sponsored by the Woodcrest Breakfast Lions will be offered on Saturday, April 25th, at the Woodcrest Vision Center, 17576 Van Buren Blvd.

J. F. Massengill, O.D., a graduate of the Ohio State School of Optometry, will perform the screening and answer your questions about computer vision.

Dr. Massengill specializes in diagnosis and treatment of computer vision syndrome and is the author of numerous journal articles.

Space is limited. If you would like to make an appointment to meet Dr. Massengill, please call 1-800-872-2020.

Example of Introductory Letter

[Letterhead]

John London
Federation Financial Services
2575 Yorba Linda Blvd
Fullerton, CA 92631

Dear Mr. London,

Allow me to introduce myself and my office. I am Dr. Eric Minteer and I am a computer vision specialist. I am new to the Fullerton area and have recently started to become active in local affairs through the Fullerton Chamber of Commerce.

There are 100 million computer users at work, with 70% of them having symptoms causing a loss of productivity. We all know that quality health care costs are soaring. Many companies are able to provide medical insurance for their employees, and some businesses are able to provide different types of vision insurance. Unfortunately, even these efforts may not be enough. Many times patients are left to bear a large financial burden on their own, particularly when computer vision care is involved.

As a way of introducing myself to the business community, I would like to extend to your company this special offer. Our office would be pleased to provide, at no additional cost to the regular examination fee, a computer vision evaluation to all of your employees and their immediate families. Additionally, we would like to add a standing 10% discount off our usual and customary fees for any additional treatment required now or in the future. We accept all major insurance plans, Visa, and MasterCard, and we can even spread payments out over several months to facilitate easy payment.

Our office is dedicated to providing quality computer vision care in an affordable manner. We specialize in compassionate patient treatment. If you have any questions or would like any additional information, please do not hesitate to call me at 879-2020.

Sincerely,

Eric Minteer, O.D.

THE DANGERS OF COMPUTER VISION SYNDROME

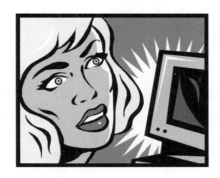

Join us for the first in a series of
FREE SEMINARS
On Thursday, April 30th—7:30 PM
Downey Public Library
11121 Brookshire Avenue, Downey
featuring
Dr. Richard Stanley

We invite you to join us for the first in a series of FREE SEMINARS featuring exciting information about you and your child's computer vision. Dr. Stanley believes building sight and creating vision are critical. Whether it be at work, school, or computer games, you and your children must be able to perform visual tasks on the computer without disabling discomfort. The evening will include a lecture and demonstration at a computer workstation. The latest specific treatments for computer-user symptoms that stem from vision problems will be the highlight of Dr. Stanley's message. You will also receive valuable and educational take-home materials for self-evaluation of your home computer workstation. Seating is limited and reservations are a must, so reserve early. We look forward to seeing you there.

<u>You Will Learn</u>

- Why vision problems are caused by computer use among children and adults
- How to identify symptoms of computer vision syndrome
- How computer vision problems can cause musculoskeletal pain

- **What can be done to correct the problems and have stress-free comfort vision on the computer**

SEATING IS LIMITED AND RESERVATIONS ARE A MUST!
RSVP (310) 862-2020

<u>What patients say about Dr. Stanley</u>

After suffering from blurry vision and headaches at work, Dr. Stanley treated me and gave me comfort and reduced stress for the first time in years! Dr. Stanley has stabilized my vision and allowed me to perform at a higher level than I ever thought possible. My 9-year-old son is doing much better in school since Dr. Stanley corrected his computer vision problem.

Example of testimonial

Dear Dr. Kame,

Computer vision care has changed my entire life. I am no longer the confused soul working double time just to figure out what others saw at first glance. It has given me freedom from the annoying and perplexing conditions that used to haunt and handicap me.

For the first time in my life, I can sit and use the computer comfortably longer than an hour. In fact, now a morning passes and I haven't even skipped a line or had double vision. My productivity has increased greatly since I am no longer plagued by losing my place and by dull nagging headaches. Surfing the Web or searching files and locating appropriate numbers is now a breeze.

Now that I'm aware of the "eyes leading the body," I have arranged my workstation to allow muscle comfort and have increased data entry speed and accuracy. I am amazed each day by the added power my new computer lenses give me. I am no longer leery of driving at night after a long day at the computer. I have improved depth perception, and I trust my judgment. Street signs come immediately into focus.

There is a small sadness when I reflect on the struggles I went through as a student and young worker trying to conquer such problems. If only computer vision treatments would have been around then, life would have been much simpler and less limiting. These thoughts of sadness are quickly forgotten and replaced with joy and excitement as I look forward to moving ahead in the future to a more fulfilled, productive life! Thank you Dr. Kame! Thanks to everyone on your team!

Julie Carlson

Index

Page numbers followed by *f* indicate figures; *t*, tables; *b*, boxes.